The Nurturing Touch at Birth:

A Labor Support Handbook

For Bonnie ~
Who was
strong & of great
courage & strength.

Polly Perez

4/11/97

Be strong and of good courage. Fear not; be not dismayed
I Chronicles 22:13–14

Life only demands from you the strength you possess.
Dag Hammarskjold

Paulina Perez

Cutting Edge Press

Cutting Edge Press
415 Bauxhall
Katy, TX 77450

Printed in the United States

Book Design and Layout by Cheryl Snedeker
Cover Design by Paulina Perez and Lori Ostapchuk
Cover Photo by Danielle Boozer
Edited by Connie Livingston

Library of Congress Cataloging in Publication Data
Paulina G. Perez
The Nurturing Touch at Birth: A Labor Support Handbook
by Paulina Perez; foreword by Phyllis Klaus, C.S.W.
Library of Congress Catalogue
97-091542
ISBN
0-9641159-8-0
1. Obstetrics-popular works 2. Natural childbirth I. Title

Cutting Edge Press books are available at special discounts for bulk purchases. For more information about how to make such purchases, please call 281-497-8894

The heart symbol that you see on the inside cover page, and throughout the book, represents the courage, bravery, boldness and tenacity that is deep inside all women. It also epitomizes the concern, compassion and loving spirit of those providing labor support to birthing women. A caring heart is at the core of their soul and the care they provide that enables the laboring mother to tap into her courage, bravery, boldness and tenacity.

For Bryan, Mark and Scott, who all live to the beat of a different drummer just like their mother

Courage is the price that life exacts for granting peace
Amelia Earhart

Acknowledgments

Don't walk in front of me,
I may not follow.
Don't walk behind me,
I may not lead.
Walk beside me
And just be my friend.
Albert Camus

To Eric, for always being at my side

To Bert and Audrey, for raising a son who is such a good man

To my parents, Theda and A.P., for providing me with a foundation of compassion and determination

To Bryan, for having the strength and perseverance to reach academic heights and longed for goals

To Mark, for being such a kind and gentle soul

To Scott, for being my "present"

To Laura, for allowing me to be her surrogate mother

To Jane, for being the sister I never had

To Michael, for having the computer knowledge without which I could not survive

To Teresa, for helping keep Cutting Edge Press running while I'm "on the road"

To Kathy, Alice Fay, David, Sue and Bill, for the magic in their hands which literally "keep me going"

To Peggy, for showing me what being a good doctor is all about

To the 600+ women in my private practice, for allowing me the privilege of attending you during your amazing birth journeys

Foreword
by
Phyllis Klaus, MFCC,CSW

In many ways, the emotional and physical support given the laboring mother is a unique art form. And just as a choreographer writes special steps for a dance, Polly Perez, in this valuable handbook, has brought together the many special positions and techniques that might be called the tricks of the trade of supporting the woman during labor and birth.

What has not always been explicit is that control of the labor is best transferred from the caregiver to the mother. As Polly Perez notes on several occasions in this book, it is the mother who must do the work of birth and one of the primary tasks of a supportive caregiver is to find out where the mother is and take her where she wants to go. The information in this book will provide both mother and caregiver more options from which to choose when approaching labor and birth. It cannot be emphasized enough that the presence of a <u>continuous</u> supportive caregiver for every mother is associated with the return to her of control over her own birth. It is exciting to appreciate how this uniquely humane approach of nurturing touch and emotional support has significantly reduced major complications of labor and permanently increased a woman's self-esteem

Phyllis Klaus
Berkeley, California

Introduction

The only thing that makes life possible is permanent, intolerable uncertainty; not knowing what comes next.
Ursula K. LeGuin

Lessons come in unexpected places and in unexplained ways. The last three years have been ones that have tried my faith and patience yet have brought me valuable life lessons and great rewards in both my personal and professional life.

I was reminded in a very abrupt way how valuable one's life partner is. Through all the trials and triumphs, I have been blessed to have Eric by my side. This was especially true while raising our three spirited sons. In February 1994 not only was I reminded how important Eric was to me, but how fierce my protective instinct was when Eric was faced with both occupational and medical hazards.

During the turmoil of the next two years, I relearned relaxation techniques long left sitting dormant and unused. Through persistence and practice, I once again realized how valuable these techniques are to all of us and most especially to laboring women. Putting these skills to use personally has added to my professional use of them too.

I experienced massage therapy on a cellular level with talented massage therapists from Texas to Missouri to Vermont. I learned in a right-brained way how important massage can be. This has had application to my professional life as a writer, lecturer, perinatal consultant, and monitrice and to my personal life. The effects of long hours at a computer, being on the road lecturing and attending birthing women has been eased by massage therapists with magic in their hands. Not only has this armed me with the knowledge to use massage skills with birthing women but to teach others about its important benefits.

Allowing myself to be nurtured has never been one of my strong suits. Allowing others to take care of me occasionally has enlightened me once again about the importance of that role. The nurturing of Sally, Kay, Pat, Sheron, Peggy, and Ana has been helpful and such a valuable lesson for me. Writing about ways to nurture laboring mothers is an offshoot of that lesson.

Observing my three sons live fulfilling, yet so very different, lives as adults has been a reward and a lesson about the value of the hard work of parenting that began with their labors and births. The lessons I learned during their births has benefited their lives as well as mine.

Trust in a professional relationship with a primary care giver was crucial to me during the last three years. Having a trusted caregiver who allowed me the time, space and unconditional support to make a very difficult decision on my own, without coercion, demonstrated to me the true beauty in the patient-physician relationship. With people being forced to move from caregiver to caregiver in the current healthcare climate, this relationship has often eroded on both sides of the patient-physician fence from one of trust to one of fear. We are seeing the dramatic impact of this throughout the healthcare system. I am blessed to have a physician who not only trusts me, but who I can trust and who demonstrates daily what being a good doctor is really all about.

Sharing on a professional level is vital to those that we care for. I have been fortunate to have colleagues like Penny, Cheri, Pat, Kelli, Phyllis , Pam and Joan who have willingly and openly shared their knowledge with me. I, in turn, am sharing that knowledge with you.

Other healthcare professionals have been generous in contributing their time and information about techniques and tips for helping laboring mothers. They include Cheri Grant, RN; Suzanna Alexander, RPT; Pat Jones, CNM; Kristi Ridd; Kelli Shelton, CNM; Penny Simkin, PT; and Teri Williams, RMT.

My collaboration with Cheryl Snedeker, Connie Livingston, Lori Ostapchuk, and Danielle Boozer was invaluable and without it, the book would not have been possible.

All of these lessons, experiences, and people have enabled me to write this book about techniques, strategies, and tools to use to help laboring women realize their strength and use their own power to give birth.

Contents

Chapter 1
What's Happening in Labor and Birth?

Even if you're on the right track,
you'll get run over if you just sit there.
Will Rogers

You must become the change that you are seeking.
Ghandi

For quite awhile, maternity care in North America has been based solely on a bio-medical model of disease treatment. We have treated pregnant women as if they were ill or diseased. They have put their trust in our ability to treat their disease called pregnancy and not in themselves. We have come to believe that pregnant women are sick and in great peril. To us, giving good care has meant rescuing the mother from this process called labor and birth. It is no wonder that we have tied women to machines, tubes and wires. It is no wonder that we have tied women to machines, tubes, and wires and told them they need drugs and anesthesia. They believed us and have asked for anesthesia in epidemic proportions. It is no wonder that women have had trouble giving birth. It is no wonder our cesarean rates have risen dramatically and new nurses and doctors are frightened about caring for maternity clients. Our disease oriented philosophy has not only changed obstetrical care but how we look at pregnant women and their families. We are all afraid. Most of the care we give is based on this fear.

Learning to Think Outside the Boundaries

Change is occurring in health care today and it is clear that we are in the midst of a health care revolution. Part of the revolution involves changing disease care to health care based on health, healing and empowerment. Those who read and use the techniques described in this book will be instrumental in adapting a new model of obstetrical care based on a bio-psychosocial model of care where the focus is on creating health and emphasizing the normalcy of pregnancy, labor and birth.

During this revolution, we are faced with an incredible opportunity and along with that comes challenges for both us and the women we care for. As we move into a new millennium, facing these challenges and taking advantages of the opportunities involved means making changes. It means taking a risk and changing how we work. Avoiding one risk often forces us into another risk. Therefore, the issue is not whether to take a risk but how to take reasonable risks. We must risk looking at birth in a new way. We must risk giving care in a new way. This has the potential to not only change women's birth experiences but society's well-being. We must change the "groupthink" about labor and birth and women's capabilities. Groupthink has been defined as the way social pressure of groups generate actions that tend to thwart consideration of alternatives. We must build bridges with others and invite views that are divergent. We must risk new ways of empowering women during pregnancy and birth. We must quit clinging to the certainty of the way we have always done things. We must risk changing! Risk is in the eye of the beholder and our fear contributes to the outcome and therefore to the risk itself. When we say things are risky what we usually mean is that it is scary to us and we feel vulnerable. Being clear about what it is that we fear is as important as determining the difference between reasonable risk and unreasonable risk. There are many risks in life and what we must decide is exactly what the specific risk is to each of us. We must decide not only what we are frightened of but what the probability of that particular outcome is. We must learn to adjust our risks by improving the odds of success. This usually involves more education, working collaboratively with others and gaining more control over the outcome. Maternity care is in transition today and we must decide between continuing the present disease-based system or changing it to a more holistic one.

The first part of any change is that which takes place within ourselves. It takes wisdom to be willing to change. We must look deep within ourselves and be self-confident so that we can handle change and encourage laboring women to do the same. Change always brings resistance to our lives which may range from mere doubts as to whether we can handle this change, to fears of losing the comfort and security of our present situation. We must quit focusing on where we work and start focusing on who we care for, as well as the skills that we possess. We must learn to use our skills in new ways or reacquaint ourselves with things we already knew but have not been using. We must ask ourselves why we are really doing the things that we do. We must ask ourselves whose needs we are satisfying; ours or the women we care for? We must stop avoiding education about new forms of health care. We must look at controversial issues and this is not easy. Supreme Court Justice William O. Douglas once said, "A person who deals with controversial issues is bound to be criticized." We must have no preconceived limitations for ourselves or laboring women. We must take the risk for our sake as well as for the sake of the pregnant women in our care.

We have the chance to help shape the maternity care of the future to better suit the needs of women, their babies, and their families. We have the opportunity to find out what families really need and provide that for them. We have the opportunity to work together more effectively and to truly collaborate with each other. Physicians, midwives, nurses and professional labor assistants can work side by side to provide comprehensive care. We can draw from each other the best that each of us has to offer instead of worrying about who does what. We can teach, nurture and motivate each other and laboring women as well. We can be prepared to make new paths and be innovative in our care. After all, there is no guaranteed linear path from the beginning to the end of labor. We must seek out alternative ways to reach our goal. We must anticipate crises along the way. All of these things will open new opportunities for both health professionals and the women they care for.

We must base our care on outcomes. We must be brave and willing to take reasonable risks. We must be willing to become results-oriented. Two skills that are shared by results-oriented people are the ability to initiate change and the ability to capitalize on change that is thrust upon them. Seize the opportunity to use the information in this book to educate yourself about new ways to care for laboring women. The future of birth is within our grasp and will come from those who excel because of all the possible changes. We must, once again, invest ourselves in pregnant women and their families. This upheaval in our maternity care system has given us an incredible opportunity to re-evaluate everything we do so that we can focus on empowering women. This in turn strengthens the family unit and therefore all of society.

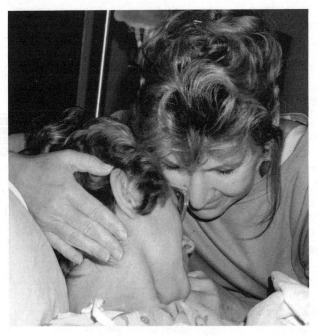

Hands are the heart's landscape.
Pope John Paul III

Chapter 2
A Caring Heart

A glad heart makes a cheerful countenance.
Proverbs 15:13

Let all that you do be done in love.
I Corinthians 13:13

Within every combination of events lies a hidden treasure,
a concealed pattern that will, with patience,
reveal itself one day as part of a
grand, inevitable, liberating design.
Alex Noble

A caring heart is the essence of supportive labor care. It is the essential ingredient in providing the type of care that enables the mother to feel safe enough to surrender to the forces of labor and allow her baby to be born. Caring comes from the heart and cannot be imitated. It is the very substance of the being of those who will use the techniques described in this handbook. This loving act called caring helps us learn about ourselves as human beings while we guide women through the birth process. Caring that comes from the heart and soul brings back humanity and kindness to the birth process that has lately been dominated by machines, tubes, and wires. Caring keeps the heart of birth alive. With a caring heart we take on the job of being a guardian of normal birth.

Caring for pregnant women during pregnancy, labor and birth requires that one of our main aims be empowerment of the mother. We gain much from seeing the mother take responsibility for herself, her baby and her birth. When we are strong, yet gentle, we teach mothers to be the same with their children and their families. When we trust and respect women, they are more apt to make good choices for themselves and their families.

The caring part of our soul rejoices when we see women grow and experience a joy they have never known. It is then that we become aware of the impact that this experience has on their lives and the lives of their families. When we hear women say immediately after pushing their baby out, "I can do anything now" our spirit is lifted and we are able to continue doing the difficult work involved in maternity care today. The impact of caring for women during labor and birth is truly about caring for them for the rest of their lives. The care we give not only impacts women and their families but society as a whole.

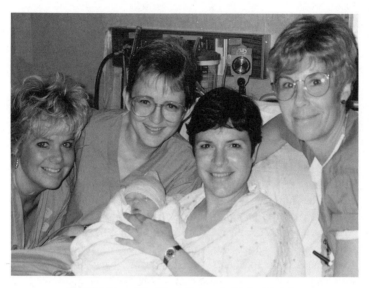

This birth team utilized the techniques in this book to help this mother have an empowering birth experience.

Chapter 3
Let's Talk About Pain

There is a way out of every dark mist over a rainbow trail.
A Navajo song

Although the world is full of suffering
it is also full of overcoming it.
Keep your face to the sunshine and you cannot see the shadow.
Helen Keller

You will forget your misery; and you will remember it
as the waters have passed away.
Your life will be brighter than the noonday;
its darkness will be like morning.
And you will have confidence because there is hope.
Job 11:10-18

A caring heart is the most essential labor support tool one can possess but there many other techniques, strategies and "tricks of the trade" to help a laboring woman mediate pain while increasing her self-confidence and ability to deal with the sensations involved in the birth process. Understanding the sources of labor pain is critical to being able to utilize labor support techniques. The sources of pain in the first stage of the labor process are the contracting uterus, the dilating cervix, pelvic pressure, ligament stretching, and compression of the roots of the lumbosacral plexus. In the second stage, the sources are stretching within the pelvis, pelvic pressure and distension of the perineum and vagina. Grantly Dick-Read published his fear-tension-pain theory in the 1930's and stated that fear increases the perception of pain by causing excitation of the sympathetic nervous system which activates contractions of the circular muscles in the uterus. This opposes the action of the upper portion of the uterine muscle causing uterine ischemia and thus pain. When assessing labor pain, it is important to consider that fear may be a factor in the pain the mother is experiencing. The mother herself may not realize that she has a fear or that it is disrupting the continuity of her labor. Until she can verbalize her fears and trepidations, her labor may progress slowly or simply fail to progress. It will help to remember the following.

When in doubt, check it out.
Consider asking the following questions:
What's going through your mind?
What do you think will help?
Tell me how you feel.
What's wrong?
Is there something that you are afraid of?

Besides the fear of pain she might express fears of those around her, the environment, the birth process, pushing, being a mother and fear for her baby. Being able to discuss these fears with her caregivers is sometimes all that is necessary for her labor to continue.

Many of the techniques in this book help block the fear-tension-pain cycle as well as stimulate endorphin (a natural pain inhibitor) production that acts by traveling to opiate receptors and by helping block reception of pain impulses. Other techniques in the book work on the gate control theory that states that the pain stimulus can be modified as it travels through the spinal cord.

The mother's beliefs and attitudes also play an important part in how she approaches the pain of labor. There are many psychological issues that have an impact on labor. These include activity vs. passivity; the ability to be uninhibited; victimization, low self-esteem and body image; a history of needing to be "rescued"; previous birth trauma or abuse (physical sexual or emotional); and awareness of fears, conflicts and concerns about birth and parenting. It is vital that we take all these factors into consideration when helping the mother cope with pain. Childbirth pain is not a hardship; it is a fact of life. Out of this pain comes growth in both a physical and emotional sense. Women are strong and capable of dealing with the pain of birth and do not need to be shielded from the realities of birth.

In order to deal with these sensations, women need realistic, yet positive, descriptions of labor pain. All those involved with childbearing women must make an effort to help women seek greater awareness of the sensations involved in birth and what they can do to cope with those sensations. Pain mediation can be accomplished by a variety of comfort measures that are non-pharmacological. Through awareness and the labor support techniques in this book, women will have an abundance of tools to deal with the pain of labor.

As mentioned, our beliefs play a crucial part in how we confront the pain of birth. In her books, Gayle Peterson discusses augmentative and diminutive beliefs and how they impact labor. Augmentative beliefs support and add to the woman's self-esteem and diminutive beliefs decrease self-esteem. Examples of augmentative beliefs are trust in the body to know how to birth; believing labor and birth are normal physiological processes; and believing women are strong and capable. Diminutive beliefs are the opposite such as disgust in bodily functions; believing birth is degrading; and believing women are weak and frail and must be rescued from the birth process.

Women's past experiences with reproduction and childbearing also greatly affect the labor process and how they deal with the pain of labor. The following situations may make it more difficult for a woman to deal with labor pain: a previous traumatic birth experience, previous sexual abuse, previous pregnancy terminations, a previous cesarean section, having relinquished a child for adoption, and a previous miscarriage, stillbirth or neonatal loss. All of these situations must be taken into account when we care for a laboring woman.

When one looks at labor support only as pain management, there is a tendency to see women as weak, frail and not capable of the task of birthing their babies without pharmacological assistance. As caregivers, we must not fear the pain of birth. Birth pain does not weaken women. Our positive attitude toward pain is the stability that laboring women long for. If we see women as victims of this process, they are more apt to see themselves in that same light. If we see them as strong and powerful and encourage them to have self-mastery in childbirth this then becomes a model for them throughout their lives. Our positive attitude about birth pain is often what the mother needs most. Our model for birth should include acknowledgment of and respect for the mind-body interaction, respect for the body's ability to birth, comprehensive education of all options, and encouragement of value based decision making.

Advantages of Natural Birth

- Natural birth is hard, but a woman's body is designed for this function. When a woman births without drugs, anesthesia or medical interventions she learns that she is strong and powerful. She learns self-confidence. She learns to trust herself, even in the face of powerful authority figures.
- Once she realizes her own strength and power, she will have a different attitude, for the rest of her life, about pain, illness, disease, fatigue, and hard or difficult situations.
- When a mother births without drugs, anesthesia, or medical interventions she will approach mothering differently. She will realize that it took hard work to bring this child into the world and it will take hard work to raise this child into an adult.
- Through all of this she will grow as a person, becoming more confident in her abilities to handle any situation that she might face and be more responsible for her own destiny.
- Natural birth allows the mother a larger range of options in terms of places to birth, positions for birth, the caregiver attending the birth and how the delivery is conducted. This allows a woman an internal locus of control (she makes decisions) versus an external locus of control (caregiver or hospital makes decisions).

Advantages of Natural Birth
- Natural birth is medically safer for mother and baby. Anesthesia and other interventions present risks to their health, which include:
Decrease in maternal blood pressure
Decrease in fetal heart tones
Decrease in uterine contractility
Increase in labor dystocia
Increase in need for pitocin augmentation
Increase in maternal temperature
Decrease in maternal ability to void
Decrease in maternal pushing ability
Increase in use of forceps for delivery
Increase in need for episiotomy and perineal trauma
Increase in need for cesarean section
Increase in fetal hypoglycemia
Increase in maternal/infant separation
Increase in breastfeeding problems
Anesthesia headache for mother
Increase in separation from family unit
Increase in post-partum back pain for mother
Nerve palsy or paralysis for mother

If mother and baby are not healthy, or progress of labor is clearly not normal, the use of drugs, anesthesia and other interventions may be justified.

It is as important to be honest about the effect medication and anesthesia has on the mother, the baby and the labor, as it is to be honest about the reality of pain during birth. Women should be told that there are side effects to mother and baby as well as the labor process when analgesia or anesthesia is used.

Intravenous medication can cause dizziness, nausea and decreased maternal blood pressure, changes in fetal heart rate patterns, depression of respiration and in the post-partum period, changes in the behavior responses of the baby. It has become commonplace for many women to request epidural anesthesia without fully understanding its effect on the labor. Side effects to the mother from epidural anesthesia involve a decrease in blood pressure, decreased ability to void, decrease in uterine contractions, increased need for oxytocin augmentation, inhibition of the bearing-down reflex, increased need for forceps or vacuum extraction, postpartum headache and, infrequently, paralysis. Side effects to the baby include changes in fetal heart rate patterns, notably bradycardia and an alteration in neurological behavior after birth such as poor muscle tone, poor sucking response, etc. The baby can also be indirectly affected by the maternal response to the anesthetic. There have been several important epidural studies done by Dr. James Thorp and colleagues. The retrospective and prospective, randomized trials have shown that continuous epidural anesthesia increases a woman's chance of cesarean section for dystocia related to the anesthesia. In fact, the prospective, controlled, randomized trial was terminated after 93 patients were entered into the study when it became clear that there was a statistically significant increase in cesarean delivery in the group receiving epidural analgesia. It was felt that it would be unethical to continue randomization.

The information contained in this book will give mothers many other options on how to deal with labor pain other than pharmacological ones. Many of these techniques for pain reduction are based on principles of neurophysiology. Through the work of physical therapist Suzanna Alexander, we understand the scientific basis for many of the pain reduction techniques described in this book. The neural receptor systems, including mechanoreceptors, chemoreceptors, and thermoreceptors all alter the mother's perception of pain. For instance, pressure on fingertips and hairless skin stimulates the mechanoreceptors called Meissner's corpuscles. These receptors transmit faster than pain thus altering the mother's perception of pain.

When assessing labor pain, it is important to consider many factors. Those factors include: immobility, fear, how rapidly the labor is progressing and the position of the baby. Being immobile often increases the mother's perception of pain. The labor is much less likely to progress well, when the mother is immobile. Changing her positions often alters her perception of pain tremendously. Fear makes any pain feel more intense. How rapidly the labor is progressing definitely alters how labor pain is perceived. When labor is rapid, more bodily work is compacted into a short space of time, thus increasing the pain felt by the mother. A precipitous labor is often very painful and the mother does not realize that it will be over quickly. It is important to let her know what is happening and that the feelings that she is experiencing are normal. Constant support is imperative and often it is helpful to consider suggesting positions to slow down the descent of the baby. Malposition of the baby often causes back pain. When the baby is in a posterior position, the mother often perceives the pain of labor predominantly in her lower back. It is important for someone with clinical skills to assess the position of the baby early in labor and encourage the mother to utilize positions and tools that encourage rotation of the baby and ease back pain.

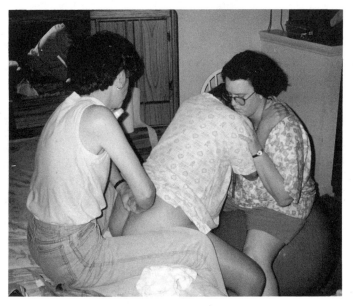

Leaning on her doula. as another labor assistant applies counterpressure, this mother's back pain is eased.

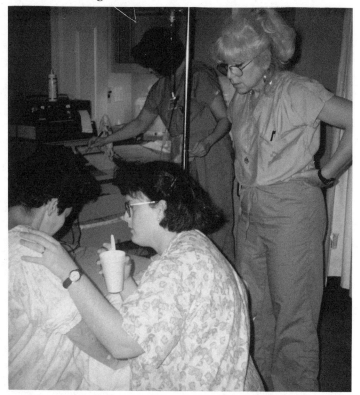

Courage is like love, it must have hope and trust for nourishment.
Napoleon

Chapter 4
Trusting Relationships and The Value of Education

In quietness and in trust shall be your strength.
Isaiah 30:15

No one is an expert on another person's life.
Eugene Gendlin

If the teacher... is indeed wise
he does not bid you to enter the house of his wisdom,
but rather leads you to the threshold of your own mind.
Kahlil Gibran

For laboring women, trust in those caring for them is a prominent aspect of labor support. It is equally important that the caregiver trust the laboring woman. As caregivers, we must get to know our clients in order to trust them. This involves taking the time to explore many issues together and giving pregnant women the time and space to make informed decisions based on the knowledge of the risks and benefits of all options. Without this knowledge of each other and mutual trust, decisions in labor by both the caregiver and the client are often based on power and coercion.

Trust is formed when all parties are equal in the relationship. Other important components of a trusting relationship are confidence, integrity, responsibility, reliability, caring and faith. When we know and truly trust the women we care for, we are then able to give them unconditional support during labor. Without mutual trust, many caregiver-client relationships have deteriorated to the point that the relationship is based on fear of each other, not trust in each other. This atmosphere makes the application of any labor support technique extremely difficult. We must be willing to confront openly, together, our concerns and fears.

Knowledge is for empowering, not overpowering. Understanding what makes a birth site safe, whether in a hospital, home or birth center, is important and should be explored in a childbirth class. Comprehensive childbirth education prepares the mother realistically for the labor and birth process and is a significant labor support tool. Suzanne Arms eloquently asks the question, "If knowledge is the best resource we can offer, in addition to loving support, what are we doing holding back information?" Therefore, childbirth education must be more than just instructions on how to get to the labor and delivery unit and what procedures to expect in labor. To be most effective, birth education should be based on a biopsychosocial model and the belief that women and their partners have inner strengths and resources which they can employ during labor and birth. Part of childbirth education is to make them aware of these inner resources through introspection, guidance, education, empowerment and support. Information about medical procedures should be prefaced by the knowledge that they should not be used routinely in labor and should be avoided in the absence of specific scientific indication for their use. This type of education desensitizes the mother to the fear of childbirth and is a very basic function of all comprehensive childbirth education. Social learning theory also shows us that the childbirth educator also acts as a role model. This is evident when she chooses videotapes that are not only informative but show realistic labor and birth situations where the mother is utilizing coping techniques.

The type of childbirth education most helpful as a labor support tool is based on principles such as the ones in *The Mother-Friendly Childbirth Initiative,* which has been ratified by the following organizations and individuals: Academy of Certified Birth Educators, American Academy of Husband-Coached Childbirth, American College of Certified Nurse Midwives, American Society of Psychoprophylaxis in Obstetrics, Perinatal Psychology and Health, Association of Women's Health, Obstetric and Neonatal Nurses, Attachment Parenting, Center for Perinatal Research & Family Support, Doulas of North America, Global Maternal/Child Health Association, Informed Parenting Midwifery Today, Midwives Alliance of North America, Midwives of Santa Cruz, National Association of

Postpartum Care Services, North American Registry of Midwives, and Wellness Associates. The initiative has as its philosophical cornerstones the following principles: normalcy of the birthing process, empowerment, autonomy, do no harm, and responsibility. These principles give rise to the following steps which support, protect, and promote mother-friendly maternity services:

- Offers all birthing mothers:
  Unrestricted access to the birth companions
  of her choice;
  Unrestricted access to continuous emotional and physical support from a skilled woman or labor support professional;
  Access to professional midwifery care.
- Provides accurate descriptive and statistical information to the public about practices and procedures for birth care, including measure of interventions and outcomes.
- Provides culturally competent care--that is, care that is sensitive and responsive to the specific beliefs, values, and customs of the mother's ethnicity and religion.
- Provides the birthing woman with the freedom to walk, move about, and assume the positions of her choice during labor and birth (unless restriction is specifically required to correct a complication) and discourages the use of the lithotomy position.
- Has clearly defined policies for:
  Collaborating and consulting throughout the perinatal period with other maternity services, including communication with the original care giver when transfer from one birth site to another is necessary.
  Linking the mother and baby to appropriate community resources, including prenatal and post-discharge follow-up and breastfeeding support.
- Does not routinely employ the following practices and procedures that are unsupported by scientific evidence, including but not limited to the following:
  shaving
  enemas
  IVs
  withholding nourishment

    early artificial rupture of membranes
    electronic fetal monitoring

- Educates staff in non-drug methods of pain relief, and does not promote the use of analgesic or anesthetic drugs not specifically required to correct a complication.
- Encourages all mothers and families, including those with sick or premature newborns or infants with congenital problems, to touch, hold, breastfeed, and care for their babies to the extent compatible with their conditions.
- Discourages non-religious circumcision of the newborn.
- Strives to achieve the WHO/UNICEF "Ten Steps of the Baby-Friendly Hospital Initiative" to promote successful breastfeeding.

    Electronic copies of this initiative may be obtained via the Internet at http://www.healthy.net/cims or by sending an e-mail message to thedocument@listserv.mcn.org, typing the word DOCUMENT in the subject line. There is also a forum web site at http://www.healthy.net/forums.htm. For more information about this initiative, its history, ways to use it, what is envisioned for it, or creative ways to support CIMS, there is a list of frequently asked questions which you may access by sending an e-mail message to:
    thedocument@listserve.mcn.org
    Put FAQ in the subject line to receive the list of questions.

Chapter 5
Communication Skills and Tools

The dream is not for the dreamer.
Tom Wolfe

You have to... learn the rules of the game.
And then you have to play it better than anyone else.
Dianne Feinstein

Being able to communicate with each other is of utmost importance if we are to work together as a team to help laboring women. Passive communication that involves no eye contact, evasive behavior and very soft voice quality often results in decreased self-esteem for the person speaking and loss of respect by those listening. It may produce a situation where someone is disliked or feels resentful. Aggressive communication denotes an attempt to gain control and a manner that is often condescending and sarcastic in tone. All but the bravest listeners are violated. When power is used in communication there are many pitfalls as it usually ends in an I-win-you lose situation. The use of power produces flight and influence; it also produces coping mechanisms in those with whom you are communicating. The best type of communication for all to use is assertive. Feelings are expressed directly and honestly and all involved have mutual respect for each other.

Those who use assertive communication are also usually creative people. Creative people can sometimes be bothersome as they question how things are done and upset firmly entrenched routines. Creative people prefer complexity to simplicity. Creativity flourishes best in a dynamic, tolerant atmosphere. Our hospital systems do not usually fit well into that definition and therefore it is imperative that creative people learn to deal with conflict. Knowing ways to deal with conflict is required for those trying to implement the use of new methods of caring for laboring women. It is fortunate that creative people are usually very flexible and are willing to shift from one approach to another when faced with a problem.

When in a situation that involves conflict or dealing with difficult people, one should work toward participative, mutual agreement or a win-win situation. This results in an increased commitment to the outcome by both parties, higher quality and quicker decisions, and warmer relationships.

It is also helpful to understand how to deal with those who are aggressive and "attack." One may initially feel confused, intimidated and overwhelmed as "attackers" tend to be abrupt, arbitrary and abusive. They often attack people, not just their behavior. Because of this, they tend to possess tremendous power in interpersonal situations. The most common reaction to them is to either back off or fight back. Both of these reactions not only rob one of the ability to deal competently with the situation but they stimulate the "attacker" to demonstrate that they are right and are in control. It is often the anger expressed by the aggressor that causes these responses. It is crucial to remember to act, not react. It also helps to think while you are feeling and feel while you are thinking.

Let attackers "run down" and, as they lose momentum, interrupt to get their attention. Don't worry about being polite and waiting for them to finish a sentence. Calling them by name and looking directly at them as you speak is beneficial. It helps if both of you are sitting down as people usually behave less aggressively when seated. Speak from your own point of view as you stand up for yourself. Comments such as "In my opinion"... and "I can see how you feel but my experience has been different..." are helpful. It is important that you not let yourself be pushed around as the "attacker" will then see you as someone to whom no attention needs to paid. Try being friendly and assertive but, above all, avoid a battle. A battle will result in a win-lose situation and someone other than the attacker will probably be on the losing end. Even when the fight is won, the battle may be lost, as it fuels the fire for later encounters.

How to Deal with Anger
Commonality
Acknowledgment
Redirect

It is beneficial to remember the acronym CAR (commonality, acknowledgment, and redirect) in situations where one must deal with anger. Anger is never appropriate in the presence of the laboring mother as her birth room should not be a battleground. Suggest stepping out into the hall. Commonality can be demonstrated by comments such as " I'm trying to help both you and my client..." and "You and I will benefit..." Try repeating what they just said to illustrate your acknowledgment. This also shows that you understand their point of view even if you don't agree with it. Distracting the angry person or gradually changing the topic may be necessary to diffuse the anger involved in the situation. The following may also be helpful when in this difficult situation.

When confronted with anger try..
Silence
Restatement
Clarification
Set limits
Gather information
Be precise and accurate
Apologize- if appropriate
Be calm
Develop solutions together

It is important to know what the laboring mother has learned prior to labor and what her expectations of the experience are. A good communication tool is a birth plan. Birth plans can also be an constructive way to avoid difficult situations in the birth room. The most effective birth plan for increasing communication between the care giver and the birthing mother is one that asks questions about wishes and expectations and avoids simply checking boxes. This type birth plan is a valuable labor support tool as it opens a dialogue between the birthing family and their caregivers resulting in shared decision making and mutual goal setting. An example of this type of birth plan is *Your Birth Plan and Your Birth* by Paulina Perez. For a copy of this birth plan, please contact the author. When reading a birth plan, learn to listen with your heart and not just your head. Listen to, not just read, what the birth plan is saying and the intention behind the words. Birth plans are labor support tools as they increase the mother's self-esteem by showing her that her preferences are respected and valued. If necessary, paraphrase what the birth plan says to assure that you understand her desires and expectations. This not only clarifies her expectations but helps establish rapport and trust.

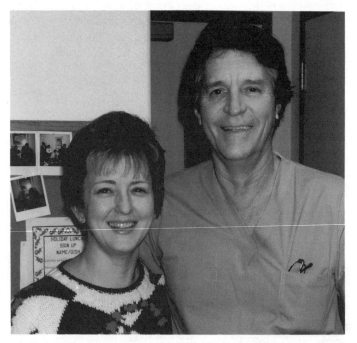

Trust and respect are integral parts of the relationship
of these two healthcare professionals.

If women are to trust their caregivers, it is important to spend the time to develop a trusting relationship. Trust is formed when we approach each other as equals. We must be honest with each other about our feelings as well as our knowledge. It is much easier to trust someone who is open and honest with you about all options available. If we expect women to trust us, we must also trust them and their ability to make the best decisions for themselves and their babies. One of the hardest things for caregivers to do is to trust and support a mother in a decision they would not personally choose. This is where taking the time to develop a trusting relationship is vital. It is also why it is more difficult for both the mother and the caregiver when they have not met each other prior to labor.

It is crucial to the outcome of the birth experience for all involved to trust and respect each other. This includes all members of the healthcare team - parents, physicians, midwives, nurses, lactation consultants, childbirth educators and professional labor assistants. It is important that the mother have the honest opinion of all involved if she is to make the best decision.

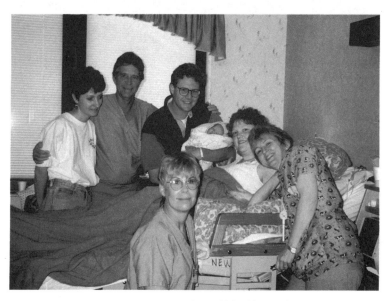

Good communication was vital to this healthcare team.

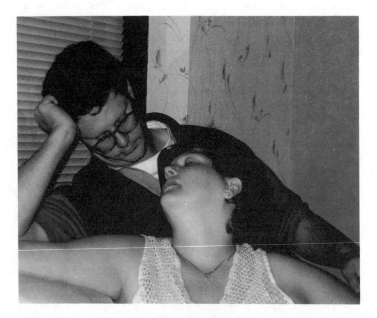

Staying relaxed is the cornerstone of
coping with labor pain.

Chapter 6
Relaxation, Affirmation, Visualization and Breathing

*A good traveler has no fixed plans
and is not intent upon arriving.*
Tao Te Ching

*Being in touch with our bodies,
or more accurately,being our bodies,
is how we know what is true.*
Harriet Goldhor Lerner

Wait patiently for what time brings.
Mahabharatam

*The aim... is to cooperate with the body
rather than regard it as a misshapen alien
or a rather unreliable but omnipresent companion.*
Jean Houston

Relaxation techniques are the cornerstones for dealing with pain as tense muscles lead to fatigue and increased pain. Relaxation works by increasing the descending inhibitory activity in the higher brain centers while it lowers heart rate, respiratory rate, blood pressure and level of blood lactates. The left brain is the center of concentration for conscious relaxation of striated muscles. Approaches to relaxation training include progressive relaxation, neuromuscular dissociation, autogenic training, meditation, and visual imagery. Progressive relaxation uses systematic tensing and relaxing of muscles. Neuromuscular dissociation asks that some muscles be tensed and others relaxed simultaneously. Autogenic training works via suggestions to the subconscious mind. Meditation encourages dwelling on an object by repeating a sound or gazing at an object while emptying the mind of all other thoughts and distractions. Visual imagery includes techniques such as visualizing a scene and is often used in combination with one of the other relaxation techniques. Be sure the mother is in a comfortable position, all body parts are supported and the environment is conducive to relaxation.

Assessing Relaxation

When assessing the woman's degree of relaxation, the "roving body check" may be used. This technique, as taught by Penny Simkin, uses touch relaxation and tone of voice to help the mother relax. Vary this technique to the needs of the mother. For instance, some mothers may prefer touch but no verbalization; others may want the reverse. Occasionally, some mothers do not want either but may use the technique by mentally scanning their own bodies. It is very important in labor to keep the muscles of the buttocks and perineum relaxed and reminders may be given to the mother to especially note those areas when roving the body. The technique for the roving body check is as follows:

Begin by asking the mother to hold her breath for a few seconds and to notice how her body feels.

Ask her to breathe out and point out the tension release as she exhales.

As the mother breathes slowly, note her rhythm and match your breathing to hers.

Use your voice in a tone and rhythm that reflects and reinforces the rhythm of her breathing.

As she breathes in, ask her to focus on a particular body part and find any tension there.

Place your hand firmly on that part creating some pressure.

As she breathes out, ask her to release any tension there.

Focus on the following body parts: shoulders, face, back of the neck, small of back, hips, buttocks, perineum, thighs and legs.

An alternative approach would be to focus only on "tension spots" and ask her to release to your touch in those areas.

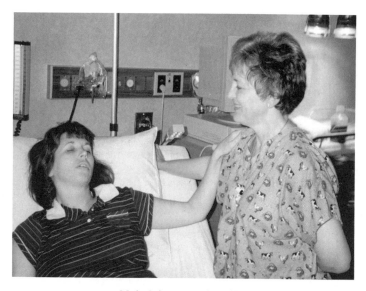

My body is strong and capable.

Affirmations

Deep within every woman is a natural intelligence that operates but the mother sometimes has to remind herself of that. Affirmations are positive statements that can be used as a labor support tool throughout labor. It is equally important for the caregivers of the mother to use affirmations as it is the mother herself. We tend to create our own reality and it helps if we have a positive attitude. Examples of positive affirmations may come in the form of religious scripture or simple statements such as the following:

> I trust my body to know how to give birth.
> I can do this contraction.
> I am strong and capable.
> My body will birth this baby.
> Labor pain is my friend.
> The contractions are a way to hug my baby.
> My baby is strong, happy and healthy.

My cervix will melt around my baby's head.
God is with me during labor, gives me strength and
holds me in his hands.

Positive affirmations are important not only to the mother but
the caregiver as well. Our care should be based on our knowledge
that birth is inherently safe, not on the fear of unexpected
outcomes.

Visualization

Visualization or guided imagery is a labor support strategy
that helps the mother develop inner awareness and control of the
body's autonomic functions as it modifies her reaction to pain. It
is used to center her, establish relaxation and is often combined
with slow deep breathing. The mother simply concentrates on
creating a picture in her mind's eye. As the words we use have a
powerful hypnotic effect, choose your words carefully. For
example, the use of the words "let go" can be substituted for the
word surrender. Using the word "surrender" can bring back
haunting memories for those with a history of sexual abuse. The
following visualizations are ones mothers have found useful
during labor and birth.

Relaxation
beach lake ocean sea shore garden waterfall special place

Breathing
breathe into the light
breathe into the pain
breathe the cervix open
breathe the pain up into your nose and out your mouth
each breath is a step up a mountain

Contractions
hugs for the baby   waves   move toward the pain

Relaxation of pelvic musculature
softening   opening   releasing   letting go

Fetal condition
happy   healthy   eager to meet parents

Fetal descent
down   putting his head on the pillow of the bag of waters
pressing the cervix open

Fetal position
seeing the baby with its head down
(this is often helpful in rotating a breech)

Cervical dilatation
the cervix melting away
the cervix moving from a turtle neck to a crew neck
a circle getting wider
mandala
bud to a blossom

Pushing
toward the sky   toward the ceiling   toward the light
seeing the color of the baby's hair   seeing the amount of hair
make a circle around the baby

Epidural Administration
make your back like a rainbow
push your back out like a mad cat

Another way for the mother to achieve relaxation and modify her reaction to pain is with the use of rhythmic breathing. Slow breathing is often the most helpful as it encourages the body to relax and "let go." This breathing pattern is done by simply breathing in through the nose and out through the mouth. Remember, it is the rhythm of the breathing that is important. Don't rush or strain; think of "letting go" with each exhalation. Use each exhalation to send tension and pain out of the body as well as to relax more deeply. Other breathing methods frequently taught in childbirth classes include light breathing, accelerated or paced breathing and a combination of breathing and light blowing. The combination light/slow breathing is often accompanied by hand signals to let the mother know how many breaths to take. Breathing may be also accompanied by an attention focusing measure such as watching the nurse, partner or labor assistant pace the breathing with her hand.

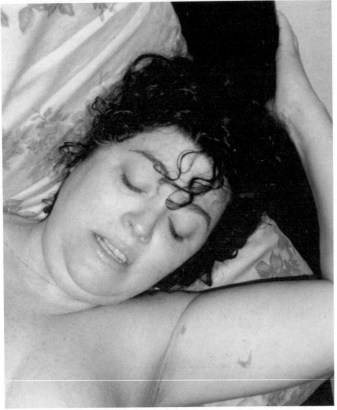

Making long low sounds helped this mother cope.

Vocalization

Vocalization often accompanies slow breathing in the form of a sign or moan. When vocalization is used, it should <u>not</u> be high pitched. The sound should come out of the mother's chest, not her throat. High-pitched sounds are frightening to the mother and have a tendency to produce tension and move the baby higher and out of the pelvis. Low, long sounds are preferable.

They resonate in the chest and sound powerful to the mother, not frightening. Encourage the mother to drop her shoulders as she makes the long, low moaning sound.

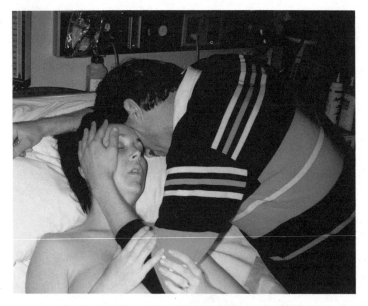

Creating an intimate atmosphere in the birth room is critical.

Chapter 7
Creating a Place in which Birth can Occur

In order to be maximally sensitive to another person,
one must be maximally sensitive to oneself.
                                        Thomas Hanna

To hear the whispered voice of another's heart
and understand unspoken words
are the talents of those lucky few
people who are precious to the world.
                                        Theresa Ann Hunt

Through the efforts of the professional labor assistant,
birth can be made safer and more satisfying.
This Special Woman can help a laboring woman
have a birth that truly goes beyond
the limits of ordinary experience.
                                        Paulina Perez

Two are better than one...
For if they fall,
one will lift up his fellow.
                                        Ecclesiastes 4:9-10

Providing the Right Atmosphere

It is critical during labor to create an intimate atmosphere for the laboring mother. This type atmosphere itself is a labor support technique as it increases descending inhibitory activity in the higher brain centers and increases the use of the limbic system. All personnel should knock lightly before entering the room and quietly enter to maintain this atmosphere. High tech environments are not conducive to relaxation and intimacy even when they are decorated beautifully. The more equipment and machines that are used, the less intimate the atmosphere regardless of the interior decorating. Dim lighting, music and attractive surroundings are nice but not essential to an intimate atmosphere. A positive attitude by all present and beliefs based on the normalcy of pregnancy and birth are essential. As caregivers, it is important for us to remember that we are privileged to be able to assist during this intimate and powerful process.

The number of people present should be chosen by the mother. For her to feel safe, she might need to surround herself with those closest to her - friends and family. All present must remember that their job is to support the mother not relate with each other.

Loud noises or voices, the entrance of people unknown to the mother and abrupt movements activate the autonomic nervous system and initiate the fight-or-flight mechanism in the mother. We should always enter the birth room as we would someone's home, with permission and respect for their space. The entire body is sensitive to sound and while the mind can be conditioned to ignore noxious sound, the body can't. These effects are below the level of conscious awareness and occur even when the mind is not consciously processing information.

A Continuous Caregiver

The undivided attention and the contance presence of someone are two of the most helpful of all the labor support techniques. This may be partly due to the Hawthorne effect. This effect is seen when someone receives what they feel is special attention from a caregiver and as a result is able to cope or perform better. Through this Hawthorne effect the mother's confidence in herself and her ability to cope increases. With increasing demands on nurses' time and the knowledge that over 50% of the nurses state they are working short-staffed, few nurses still have the privilege of being with the mother one-on-one continuously throughout labor and birth. Therefore, a new member of the healthcare team is often incorporated in the form of a professional labor assistant. The doula or monitrice is trained in labor support techniques and stays with the mother continuously providing emotional and physical support. Current research shows us that with the continuous emotional and physical support of a labor assistant there can be a 50% reduction in overall cesarean rate, a 25% reduction in length of labor, a 40% reduction in oxytocin use, a

30% reduction in the use of pain medication, a 40% reduction in the use of forceps, and a 60% reduction in the request for epidural anesthesia. For more information on this role, read *Special Women: The Role of the Professional Labor Assistant* by Paulina Perez and *Mothering the Mother* by Klaus, Klaus and Kennell.

Supporting the Laboring Mother Emotionally

Emotional support strategies are the building blocks of labor support. They include: undivided attention, expressions of caring, belief in the mother's ability to birth, attention focusing, establishing a ritual, reassurance, and verbal reminders. In the work of Nichols and Hummenick, one learns that the gate control theory is felt to work through the descending pathway of the nervous system as well as the ascending pathway which may account for the effectiveness of many cognitive strategies such as focusing, music, mental activity and rhythmic breathing. These strategies involve the mother's mind in mental activities other than the pain she is experiencing. This may interfere with the transmission of painful sensations or their interpretation.

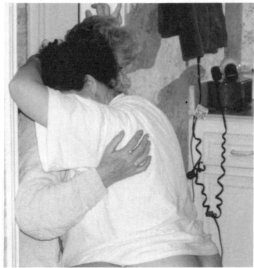

When labor is chaotic and confusing, having someone touch and hold the mother can support her emotionally.

Mental Activity

Mental activity during a contraction is another way of modifying the mother's reaction to pain. This may occur in many forms such as chanting, singing songs, repeating scriptures, rhymes, mantras, numbers, breaths or colors. Actually, the list is endless as women are very creative at developing mental activities to help themselves during labor. A visual focal point often provides another attention focusing comfort measure. Eye contact with her partner, nurse, midwife or labor assistant may be preferred by the mother or simply gazing at a picture. Attention focusing techniques also include, music, voice, and touch and are usually more effective than distraction techniques.

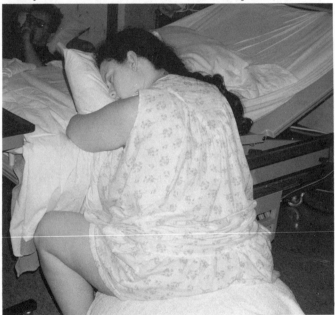

Sitting on the birth ball is part of this
mother's birth ritual.

Birth Rituals

Any of a number of techniques may be used by the mother as a birth ritual. This repetitive rite is a simple way of coping with the contraction. She may want to walk in a certain pattern repeatedly or hold the same person's hand with each contraction. If the mother is using a visual focal point, be sure no one obstructs her view of it. If she uses self talk or repeats verses, do not interrupt her. She may want to hear the exact same piece of music over and over. She may want certain scriptures repeated to her at certain times. The mother might choose the same midwife or labor assistant with each birth as a way of establishing harmony in her environment. She may wear the same piece of clothing for each of her births as part of her ritual. All of these items and patterns are the mother's way of establishing some sense of order in a fairly chaotic process.

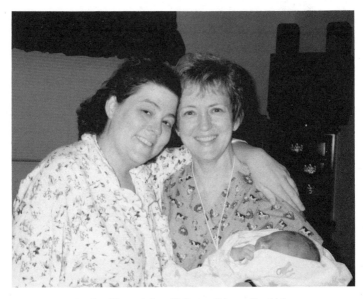

Having this monitrice with her at all three of her births
was part of this mother's birth ritual.

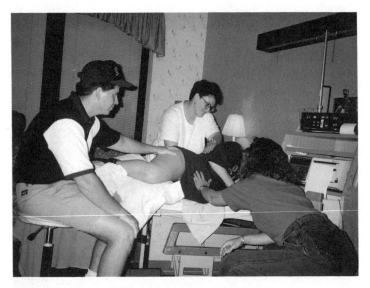

Massage touches the body and spirit.

Chapter 8
Touch and Massage

Often the hands will solve a mystery
that the intellect has struggled with in vain.
C.G. Jung

When you touch a body, you touch the whole person,
the intellect, the spirit, and the emotions.
Jane Harrington

Massage is a coping strategy that increases transmission of innocuous impulses and reduces painful stimuli. Simply put, it is a way of speaking nonverbally to the right brain. Muscles are part of the neuro-muscular-skeletal system and for any purposeful action to be performed one of these three systems must be involved. The muscular system is a vast interlacing of tissue fibers. Keeping other muscles relaxed while the uterine muscle does its work during labor enhances the progress of labor.
Massage releases toxins from the muscles and keeps the muscles oxygenated.
Always ask the mother's permission before you touch her. Massage strokes should be long, slow and directed outward. Be sure your hands are warm before doing massage techniques. Center yourself by concentrating on your own slow, relaxed breathing. Keep your fingers together when you knead or stroke the tissue. Always maintain constant physical contact and make your movements rhythmic and smooth. Moving your whole body helps develop a nice rhythm. **Never hurry when doing massage.** Use oil or lotion to decrease friction. Some massage oils are scented for the aromatherapy effect. The Happy Massage Oil™ has two different types that utilize aromatherapy. The naturally uplifting oil has extracts of melon and cucumber to stimulate the senses by refreshing. The naturally soothing oil has essential oils of bergamot, vanilla and rose wood to calm and relax the mother. One can make their own massage oil by blending an essential oil into a base oil. When applying oil, put it

in your hands first. Slowly move your hands together or stroke with one at a time. Use the weight of your body to apply the needed pressure. If you rely strictly on arm pressure, you will tire easily. Feel the contours of the muscle as you massage.

Effleurage is a long, stroking movement used in massage and may be done by mother herself as light, rhythmic stroking on her lower abdomen in either a circular or side-to-side motion. Typically, effleurage begins with light stroking which can be replaced with short strokes of greater pressure.

A type of massage welcomed by many mothers is gently brushing her hair. One might also try giving her a neck and head massage. A technique for a head and neck massage is as follows:

> Stand behind the mother and put your hands on her shoulders.
>
> Massage the muscles that run along her neck into her shoulders.
>
> Make your first strokes long and light and then begin using the weight of your body to apply more pressure.
>
> Move your hands up to the sides of her forehead and gently rub at her temples.
>
> As you move up to her scalp, spread your fingers and massage her scalp as if you were shampooing her hair. Do this until you can feel the scalp gently move back and forth on her skull.

In labor, many mothers may welcome hand or foot massage when they prefer not to be touched elsewhere. The following technique may be used for foot massage:

Hold the foot firmly in both hands.

Apply pressure with the thumbs on the ball of the foot at the top center of the instep.

Massage the top of the foot by kneading.

Pull on the toes, one at a time, and rotate them several times in each direction.

You might also want to try fast hand-over-hand circulation strokes.

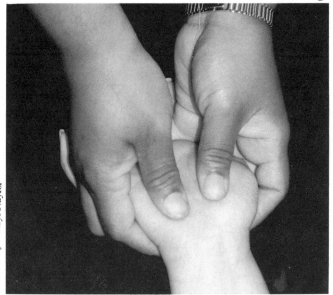

Photo by Cheryl Naylor

There are two hand massage techniques that are especially productive during labor. The techniques are as follows:

> With the mother's hand palm down, grasp her hand with your thumbs on the top of her hand and your fingers on her palms.
>
> Stroke the top of her hand from the center outward.
>
> While many mothers prefer firm pressure always check with the mother to be sure of the degree of pressure that she prefers.
>
> Wrap your fingers around the back of the hand for support and grasp the palm side with the flat surface of both thumbs.
>
> Use your whole thumb to knead the hand, not just your finger tips.
>
> Concentrate on the fleshy part of the hand but firmly move your thumbs around so that the entire surface of the hand is covered.
>
> Next, slowly stroke each finger once from the base to the tip.
>
> You might also pull lightly on each finger in a downward direction.

> With the mother's left-hand palm upward, insert the last two fingers of your left hand under the last two fingers of her hand as you insert the last two fingers of your hand under the ringer finger and thumb of her hand.
>
> Your fingers are all on the top of her hand and your thumbs are used to stroke the palm as you stretch it open.

An alternative movement is simply to "walk down her palm" with your thumbs.

It is most important that the mother keep her pelvis relaxed. With her permission, massage her thighs and buttocks to keep her pelvis and perineum relaxed. You may use the following technique:

> Stand behind the mother and give the muscles of the buttocks firm stroking or kneading.
>
> Move to a position in front of the mother and knead the big muscles in the thighs as well as using stroking movements.

Although these techniques may be difficult to learn they are welcomed by the laboring mother. Remember that massage should feel good; check with the mother frequently about the amount of pressure she prefers. You may find she will ask you to increase the pressure as you use the technique. Massage tools such as the Happy Massager™ are often extremely helpful for those with no experience doing massage.

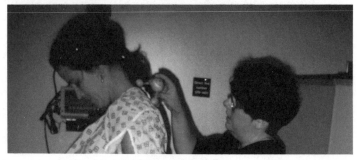

The doula uses the Happy Massager™ to enhance the mother's relaxation.

Chapter 9
Healing Arts Modalities for Use with the Laboring Woman

After the verb to love,
to help is the most beautiful verb in the world.
Countess Bertha von Suthen

the violets in the mountains
can break rocks
if we believe in them
and allow them to grow
Unknown author

Aromatherapy

Aromatherapy is another labor support strategy that uses essential oils extracted from aromatic plants to enhance or restore well being. Its use dates back to the time of Hippocrates, the father of medicine, and is both effective and enjoyable to use. Hippocrates recommended a daily bath or massage with essential oils as part of the way to health. As the aroma of the essential oils is picked up by the fine hairs in the nose and via nerve impulses transferred to the limbic system which controls memory and emotion. Essential oils have complex molecular structures. A French chemist, Rene-Maurice Gattefosse, was the first to use the name aromatherapy. Many hospitals in both Europe and North America are now encouraging the use of aromatherapy for those in their institutions. Aromatherapy works directly on the limbic and olfactory systems. The limbic system is closely connected with the pituitary gland which affects hormonal function. Essential oils may be added to baths, foot baths, rinses after a bath, compresses, massage, and vaporization. When using essential oils in baths, the benefit is reaped from inhaling the oil as well as absorbing it through the skin. Never apply undiluted essential oil onto the skin. Research studies are presently being conducted in both North America and Britain on olfaction and the effects of oils. Different oils have different effects. Essential oils should be kept away from the eyes and out of reach of children and are never to be taken internally.

Aromatherapy is a very pleasurable way to relieve stress during labor and birth. One way to use essential oils in the birthing suite is to put a few drops of essential oil mixed in water in a squirt dispenser and spray the room. For relaxation, you might use neroli, ylang-ylang, lavender, or rose. If the mother's spirits need to be lifted or revived, you might try rosemary, geranium, juniper, or eucalyptus. Another way to use aromatherapy during labor or birth is to put a few drops of essential oil on a handkerchief or face cloth and put that close to the mother's head. For help with pain, clary sage can be added to the massage oil used on the mother's lower abdomen or back. One can also use compresses with essential oil in those same areas.

Aromatherapy for CareGivers

A massage or bath with rosemary oil is excellent to revive tired muscles. For care givers who must be on their feet most of the day, a foot bath with juniper, rosemary and lavender can be very helpful at the end of a long day. One might also massage a few drops of lavender or rosemary into your temples.

The Value of Music

Music therapy is another important coping tool. Music and sound can help bring a greater degree of both physical and psychological balance. The most important element in choosing music for use during birth is that the mother be the one to choose the music that is right for her. Hospital birthing units and birth centers often keep a selection of tapes or CD's on the unit for those who do not bring their own music. Often nurses on the unit contribute their favorite music and families leave music to be used by others.

Music activates the right brain which mediates pain better than the left brain and stimulates the autonomic nervous system. Because music is nonverbal, it can move through the auditory cortex directly to the center of emotional responses in the limbic system. Music helps by controlling somatic and autonomic activity of the brain and it causes physical responses which include a change in heart rate, circulation and respiratory activity as well as psychological responses. The birth site should be furnished with the equipment needed to utilize music therapy during labor. If this is not possible, encourage all laboring women to bring their own CD's or tapes.

Music is even more beneficial when combined with imagery or visualization for relaxation. Different types of music can be employed at various times during labor. Following are some suggestions for use of music during the labor and birth process.

For relaxation, choose music with a 3/4 or 4/4 tempo played
   softly
For active labor, choose music with a 4/4 distinct slow beat with
   moderate intensity or a 4/4 moderately fast tempo with
   moderate intensity
For pushing, choose music with a 4/4 distinct driving
   moderatebeat loudly

Possible music selections for labor and birth are listed below.

Classical

Relax with the Classics	Vol. 1 Largo Vol. 2 Adagio
	Vol. 3 Pastorale Vol. 4 Andante
Stress Busters	This contains many classical
	pieces played at 60 beats per
	minute (a good resting heart rate)
Jean Pierre Rampal	Four Centuries of the Flute
Bach	Brandenburg Concerto # 2
	First Movement
	Brandenburg Concerto #4
	Last Movement
	Brandenburg Concerto # 5
	First Movement
	Jesu, Joy of Man's Desiring
	Ave Maria
Beethoven	Ode to Joy
Handel	Water Music
Mozart	Piano Concerto #21 in C Major

	Especially the second movement and when played by Giza Arda and the Camerata Academia des Salzburg Mozarteums
Pachelbel	Canon in D
Ravel	Daphnis and Chloe Suite #2
Schubert	Trout Quintet
	Especially the fourth movement and when played by the Budapest String Quartet
Vivaldi	Concerto for Two Guitars and Orchestra in D Major
	The Four Seasons

Traditional/Religious/New Age

Somewhere in Time soundtrack

Fisherfolk Sing Psalms	Joy in the Morning
Philip El Cano	Rain Dance (this was composed for use during his wife's labor)
	Cloud Dancers
Enya	Watermark
Fred Schwartz	Transitions
George Winston	Winter into Spring
	Autumn
	December
Kitaro	Numerous works
Magical Strings	Above the Tower
Michael Jones	Wind and Whispers
	Sunscapes
Steven Halpern	Spectrum Suite
	Comfort Zone
	Starborn Suite
	Sweet Baby Dreams
Zamfir	Pan Flute Music
John Tesh	Numerous selections

White Noise

Nature Recordings	The Sea
Ryko	Waterfall from the series A Day on Cape Cod
Environments	Slow Ocean
Nature's Journey	Gentle Island Surf (a combination of music & nature sounds)
Listener's Choice	Spectacular Thunderstorms (a blend of music & nature sounds)

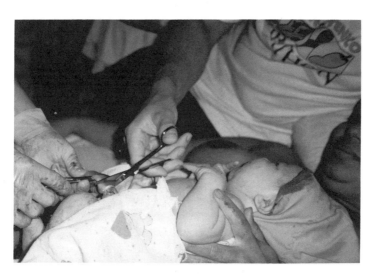

Music, chosen by the parents, played as this father
cut his son's umbilical cord.

Therapeutic Use of Water in Labor and Birth

The use of hydrotherapy is extremely helpful for pain relief during labor. Two things happen when the body is immersed in water. The thermal effect of the water relaxes the muscles and softens all the tissues and the buoyancy relieves stress on the entire system and promotes rest. Hydrostatic pressure is the second effect of immersion on the body in water. The water puts steady deep pressure on the body that fires off all the pressure receptors that say to the body, "OK, relax." Bathing is a psychological leisure time activity most people associate with feeling good. Resting in a tub, shower or Jacuzzi diminishes production of catecholamines. For the mother experiencing the irritation and discomfort of prodromal labor, the tub or Jacuzzi may be a lifesaver. Being buoyant in the water often causes the erratic and sometimes ineffective contractions to space out so the mother may rest. Being in the tub may be the only way the mother feels comfortable. It is important when using hydrotherapy to make sure that the mother stays hydrated by sipping juice, water, or electrolyte balanced drinks constantly.

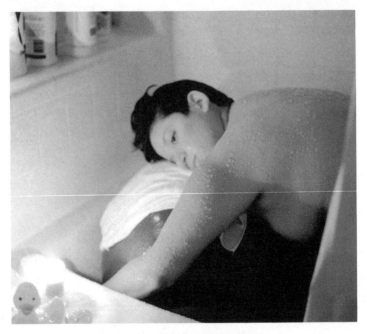

This mother chose the bath, shower, and birth ball
to help her cope with prodromal labor

The spray of a shower soothes the sacral pain felt by mothers experiencing back labor. Nurses frequently comment that putting a mother in the tub is equal to a dose of a narcotic but with no side effects. Since many women find laboring in water extremely helpful in coping with labor pain it is not surprising to find that many birth sites are incorporating tubs and Jacuzzis in their pain management care plans. The pain of labor is eased by having the mother use the tub, Jacuzzi or shower frequently throughout labor. Combining hydrotherapy with other labor support tools and strategies is also beneficial. For back labor, the mother might lean over a birthing ball in the tub as the shower sprays beats on her lower back. **The water in the tub, Jacuzzi or shower should never be above 100 degrees.**

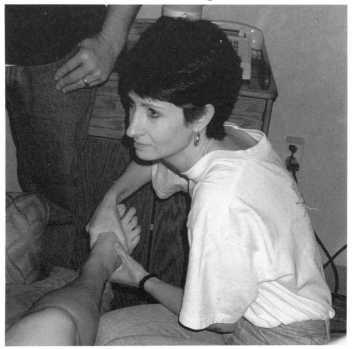

Foot massage and acupressure are used by this labor assistant
to help the mother.

Acupressure

Acupressure is a very versatile treatment that evolved from the same Oriental roots as shiatsu and acupuncture. Acupressure uses finger pressure on acupuncture points to treat imbalances of the body energy called Qi. Oriental philosophy tells us this vital energy is what keeps our bodies functioning. The treatment works by pressing on specific points close to the surface of the skin that are located along the energy meridians called channels of Qi. When giving acupressure both giver and the receiver of acupressure should wear comfortable, loose clothing. Some acupressure therapists feel that is it is better if there is a thin layer of clothing on the recipient so that the therapists attention remains with the subtle energy flow and not on the feeling and texture of the skin.

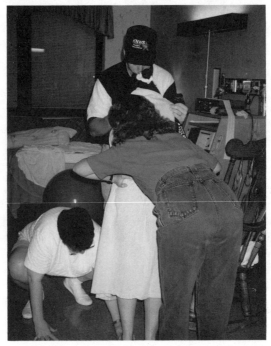

Acupressure techniques can help a labor progress more
efficiently and be less painful.

You can tell when you've located an acupressure point as it is sensitive to pressure. The following is general information about the use of acupressure in labor. Various finger manipulation techniques are used but small circular motions and steady deep pressure are the most common. Press at these points throughout a contraction. The literature is variable about the length of time you hold the pressure with the range being 10 seconds to 3 minutes, whichever the mother prefers. A reactive hyperemia may be noticed when the pressure is removed. Acupressure points that help labor are spleen 6, large intestine 4, bladder 60 and bladder 67.

Spleen 6 is located four fingers from the top of the ankle on the inside of the leg behind the shin bone toward the back of the leg.

Large intestine 4 is also known as the Ho-ku point and is found on the back of each hand in the webbing between the thumb and index finger, one inch from the edge of the webbing.

Bladder 60 is on the outside of the foot in the depression just to the back of the ankle, halfway between the Achilles tendon and the knob of the ankle bone.

Bladder 67 is one tenth of an inch to the outside of the bottom corner of the small toenail.

Most books on acupressure caution against using Large Intestine 4, Bladder 60 and Spleen 6 during pregnancy prior to labor as acupressure on these areas may produce contractions.

There are tools that can be used that utilize acupressure points. An eye pillow filled with natural ingredients that is placed over the eyes gently massages the acupressure points to aid in relaxation. Some eye pillows are also lightly scented for the Aromatherapy effect. The Happy Massager™ can also be used to stimulate acupressure points. For more detailed information contact an experienced acupressure therapist in your area.

Reflexology

Reflexology is a treatment used to normalize the body's functioning. Its use is over 4,000 years old and paintings in tombs in Egypt depict reflexology treatments being given. Its documented use dates as far back as the 4th century BC in China by Dr. Wang-Wei. This therapy was brought to North America in the early 19th century by physician who worked in London England, as well as Boston, Massachusetts and Hartford, Connecticut. Gentle pressure is applied to various points on the feet or hands that correspond to different body systems. The aim is to bring normal physiological functioning to those systems. Reflexology can be used in labor and birth to help relieve stress. There is an area on the foot that helps with the sciatic area which is sometimes bothersome to laboring women. The following technique can be utilized.

> Support the right foot with your hand and use the index and third fingers of the left hand to work up the area just behind the ankle about 3 inches. This may be repeated two or three times. Reverse your hands for the left foot.

There is also a tool that can be used to stimulate the feet. The Happy Roller™ massages the reflexology points of the feet. These points affect the entire body and help improve circulation, relieve stress and balance the body's energy.

According to hand reflexology theory, grasping combs so that they press on the pressure points of each hand on the tips of fingers, thumbs and the upper part of the palm is helpful in mediating pain. This is similar to grasping someone's hand. The reflexology theory is that pressure on the balls of the hands and the mid fingertips facilitates soothe, rapid and less painful contractions of the uterus. The mother grasps a comb in each hand so that the tines of the comb press on the pressure points mentioned and then she squeezes tightly during contractions. This can also be accomplished by grasping small massage tools.

The Mini Massager™ can be squeezed instead of combs. Some mothers maximize the reflexology effect by grasping two massagers, one in each hand. Another theory about why this works is the analgesia that it gives is due to it being a counter irritant.

Therapeutic Touch

Therapeutic touch uses the natural energy field of the caregiver's hand to assess the energy field of the mother for cues to differences in quality of energy flow. It is the direction of life energy from the caregiver to the mother. Much of the research in this field has been done by a nurse, Dr. Dolores Krieger. This therapeutic use of hands appears to be a universal act and written history of it goes back some 5,000 years. The caregiver must have the intention of healing, must be motivated to help the mother, and must have knowledge of the techniques used in therapeutic touch. In order to use therapeutic touch one must be in touch with their feelings. The caregiver must center themselves before beginning to use this modality. Therapeutic touch processes involve working in parallel. Dr. Kreiger explains that the healer (caregiver) remains on center throughout the therapeutic touch session, even while engaging in the healing techniques. This ability to tune in, not out, and to be extremely sensitive is part of the basis of therapeutic touch. For in-depth information on this method, consult Dr. Krieger's books listed at the end of this book.

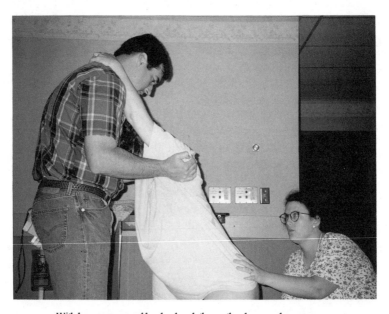

With her arms around her husband, the mother leans and sways.

Chapter 10
Innovative Strategies and Techniques

For wisdom will enter your heart,
knowledge will be pleasant to your soul.
Proverbs 2:10

When love and skill work together, expect a masterpiece.
John Ruskin

Slow Dancing

Slow dancing is a labor support technique that combines the upright position, rhythmic movement, relaxation, touch and often counterpressure. The mother stands with her arms around her partner, midwife, nurse, or labor assistant and leans and sways. This movement helps in the rotation of the fetus in a posterior presentation and helps realign a fetus that is presenting in an asynclitic position as gravity aids descent. This technique may be used with or without music.

Hot and Cold

Application of heat or cold are both helpful to the laboring woman. Heat increases the extensibility of tissue as the collagen tissue can actually become longer. Heat also clears metabolites and toxins from the body. Hot packs might be available from the physical therapy department at the hospital but a very convenient form of moist heat is the hot rice pack or **Hot Sox.** This lavender scented hot rice pack is made by a practicing professional labor assistant. It is the largest one on the market and is perfect for use on the lower abdomen, shoulders or low back. Hot packs can be made on the spot by heating a damp towel in the microwave and cover it with a hospital chux pad. **When using hot packs, the temperature of the hot pack should never be too hot to hold in**

one's hand. The application of cold often offers more relief for acute back pain than heat. One might use a surgical glove filled with ice, an ice bag, a cold beverage can, an ice filled rolling pin or an ice wrap made for this purpose. The ice wrap is a large pliable, reusable ice pack with stretchable straps and a Velcro closure. It may be used while the mother is ambulating or in any labor position. For back pain, it is often best to use the application of cold first. Cold actually alters the activity of peripheral nerves that allow the muscles to relax. Cold decreases the firing, excitation and conduction of pain neurons. It also has an anesthetic effect. Always be sure the mother is warm before applying a cold pack. Maximum effect from cold is reached within 20-30 minutes. **Place at least one layer of clothing under the cold pack; never apply cold packs directly to the skin.** Alternating heat and cold helps avoid habituation to the sensations, thus allowing the techniques to be effective for a longer length of time.

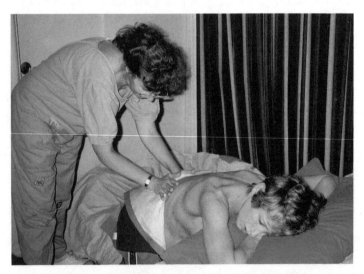

The application of cold via this ice wrap allows the mother to move about while still bringing benefits to back labor .

Double Hip Squeeze

Another support strategy helpful for those experiencing back labor is the double hip squeeze. This approach is tricky to learn but is well worth the effort as mothers find it mediates the pain of back labor very effectively. The technique is demonstrated in the video *Comfort Measures for Labor* with Penny Simkin and *Special Women: How a Labor Assistant Makes Birth Safer, More Satisfying and Less Costly* with Paulina Perez, RN   The technique is as follows:

Locate the mother's iliac crest on each side.
Mentally picture a V from the crests to the coccyx.
The spots for hand placement are below and outside the midline of each side of the V.
Press in and upward at those spots during a contraction.
Ask the mother how much pressure is best.

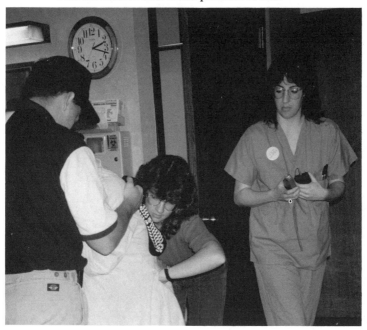

The double hip squeeze is a technique that is very helpful for back labor.

An alternatives to press directly on the iliac crests in the same up and inward motion. Try both techniques and use the one the mother feels is best for her. This technique can be tiring to the person doing it but is ever so helpful to the mother. Teri Williams has modified this technique in the following manner.

> With the mother on her hands and knees on the floor, straddle your legs over her.
> With your legs on either side of the mother push inward and forward with your knees as you put pressure on her lower back with your hand.

Knee Press

The knee press is another helpful technique for back pain. It can be used with the mother sitting in a chair with good back support or when she is side lying. When the mother is sitting in a chair with good back support or a small pillow at her lower back, apply pressure just below each knee cap in a forward motion throughout the contraction. To avoid this technique becoming tiring, use your body weight to apply the pressure by leaning forward. When the mother is in a side lying position, one person can apply the knee pressure and another applies pressure on the lower back.

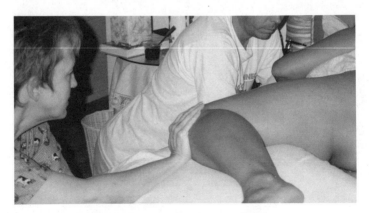

The knee press can also be done while the mother is
lying on her side.

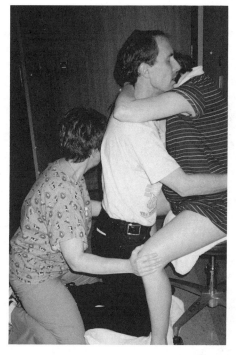

As the mother sits on a stool with her back against the wall, the knee press helps with low back pain.

Subcutaneous Injections of Sterile Water

Subcutaneous intracutaneous injections of sterile water at four sites in the lower back have been proven to help relieve the back pain experienced by approximately one third of laboring women. Researchers reporting in the *American Journal of Obstetrics and Gynecology* and the journal *Pain* point out that this stimulates other nerve endings in the skin of the lower back and works either by the gate control theory or through the release of endorphins. It seems to provide pain relief while avoiding the motor block and side effects that of epidural anesthesia. The researchers report that this technique achieves rapid, dramatic and often complete relief of back pain and that the analgesic effect lasts sixty to ninety minutes. For further information on this pain relieving technique consult "Intracutaneous sterile water for back pain in labour" in *Canadian Family Physician*, Vol. 40, October 1994. This technique is demonstrated in the video *Intracutaneous Injection of Sterile Water for Relief of Low Back Pain in Labour* by J.L. Reynolds, MD.

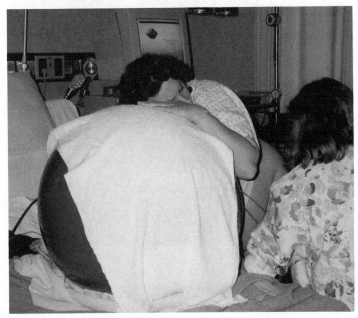

Leaning on the birth ball is not only relaxing, but takes
advantage of gravity and pelvic mobility.

The Gymnastik Birth Ball

The birth ball is a physical therapy ball that not only facilitates physiologic positions for labor but is an essential comfort tool for pregnant women. This ball is a professional physical therapy ball and not a toy as are the ones often found in children's stores. The ball should be large enough to sit on with legs bent at a 90-degree angle. The size that is best for use with laboring mothers is usually the 65cm ball. The Gymnastik birth ball is ribbed to prevent it from sliding. It is easily cleaned with soap and water or solutions used to wipe down hospital beds and equipment. Inflate the ball so it is firm. The video guide for

Comfort Measures for Childbirth with Penny Simkin states that the ball will hold up to 300 pounds. Keep sharp objects away from the ball and it is best not to store it in temperatures warmer than 80 degrees F.

Mothers are encouraged to hold the ball with their hand as they sit down on it with their feet flat on the floor and about two feet apart to give them a stable base. If the mother is concerned about feeling stable, have her partner, professional labor assistant, nurse or midwife stand behind her until she feels stable. The ball can be used in conjunction with both external and internal electronic fetal monitoring. Its use is demonstrated by Paulina Perez, Penny Simkin, Cheri Grant and other trainers in doula workshops throughout North America.

This versatile ball has a myriad of uses. It encourages pelvic mobility as it allows the mother the freedom to rock her pelvis, change her position and shift her weight for comfort. Mothers report that the ball is valuable in the last month of pregnancy as they find it easier than a chair or couch to get up and down from. In labor, it encourages fetal descent as the mother remains sitting in an upright posture taking advantage of gravity. Sitting on the ball helps keep the fetus well aligned in the pelvis. It encourages pelvic relaxation by conforming to her body similar to a water mattress as it provides perineal support without undue pressure. Sitting on warm compresses on the ball will maximize perineal relaxation. As the mother sits on it, the ball also encourages rhythmic movement as the mother sways or rocks back and forth. Sitting on the ball while leaning over the bed gives the mother the pelvic mobility that she is unable to have while sitting on a chair. The ball may also be used as a support while squatting. This encourages fetal descent while the squatting position widens the pelvic outlet to its maximum. The ball may find its most important use in the care of the mother with a fetus in the persistent posterior position. Having the mother lean over the ball while on her hands and knees gives her good pelvic mobility as well as uses gravity to encourage the largest and heaviest part of the baby's body to rotate. Kneeling and leaning over the ball assists in rotation of the baby to the anterior. As the mother's weight is totally supported by the birth ball, she is able to stay in the critical hands and knees position for an extended length of time. Normally the mother is only able to maintain this position for a short interval as it causes carpal tunnel syndrome by putting excess strain on her wrists and hands and is tiring as she must support her entire body weight. The use of the ball has saved more than a few mothers from a cesarean section for failure to progress.

The ball may also be used following birth for both calming a fussy baby and post-partum exercises. With a fussy baby, the mother sits on the ball and sways or bounces slightly while patting the baby. Mothers also report that they have used it for colic by placing the baby on its stomach on it; the pressure on the baby's abdomen seems to help. The mother should always steady the ball when the baby is on it. Exercises using the ball in the postpartum period can help firm and tone the hip and buttocks, inner and outer thighs and abdomen. Postpartum exercises for the lower body are explained in detail in *The Body Ball Book.*

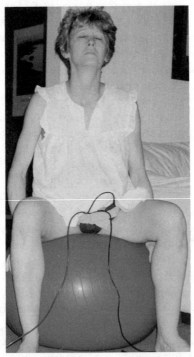

The birth ball can be used in conjunction with either external or internal electronic fetal monitoring.

The Lunge

The human body is a wonderful work of art and can be used very effectively to help rotate a baby in the persistent posterior position. The lunge is one way to use the body to help the baby rotate. The nurse, midwife or physician will be able to tell via Leopold's maneuver which side the baby's back is on. The mother should lunge to that side. If the position of the baby is unknown to the mother, have her try lunging to both sides and choose which feels more comfortable. Directions for doing the lunge are as follows:

> Stand next to an arm chair.
>
> Place one foot on the chair with the knee and foot pointing to the side while you remain facing forward.
>
> Slowly lean or "lunge" sideways toward the chair so that you bend the knee of the leg that is placed on the chair.
>
> You will feel the stretch on the inside of both thighs.
>
> Stay in the lunge position to the count of 8 before returning upright.
>
> Repeat during or in between contractions.

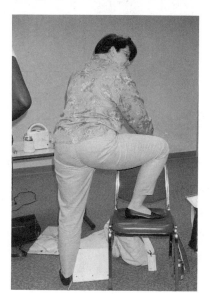

The lunge helps rotate a baby in the posterior or asynclitic position.

The Dangle

The dangle is a technique similar to a standing squat that will help the baby to descend into the mother's pelvis. Someone sits on a high counter with their legs far apart. The mother backs up and stands between their legs. When the contraction starts, the mother dangles by taking all of her weight off her feet. She is supported by her arms and shoulders over the caregiver's thighs. The technique helps lower the baby into the pelvis by utilizing gravity and encouraging relaxation of pelvic muscles. This support strategy is extremely easy to utilize with a hospital birth bed by removing the end of the bed, using the foot rests for support and increasing the height of the bed. This technique is often combined with pushing for use in the second stage of labor.

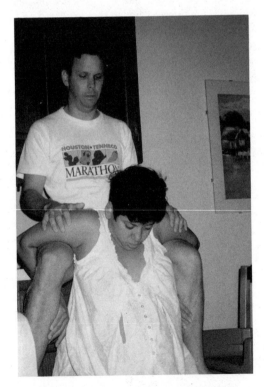

The dangle helped the baby descend into the pelvis.

Pelvic Circles and Abdominal Lift

Whether it is to encourage descent or rotation of the baby, pelvic movement is often the key. Encourage the mother to utilize positions and products that promote pelvic mobility. As stated previously, the birth ball is very effective. Among the myriad ways to promote pelvic mobility are slow dancing, the lunge, the dangle, pelvic rocking and pelvic circles. Pelvic circles are done by having the mother stand with her arms around someone's neck and making circular movements with her hips during contractions. The key is not to break the circle but keep the movement constant. This uses the forces of the contraction and the pelvic movement to encourage the fetus to rotate as well as descend. This technique is helpful for mothers with babies in the persistent posterior or asynclitic position. Another technique that is helpful for the twenty-five percent of babies that are in the persistent posterior position is the abdominal lift. This technique is simple to accomplish. The mother lifts her abdomen with her hands while having a contraction. Perinatal nurse and doula Cheri Grant calls this technique the apron lift.

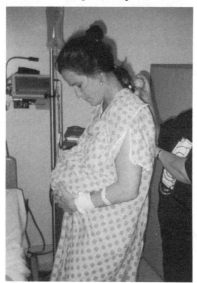

The mother uses the apron lift to help rotate her baby from the persistent posterior position.

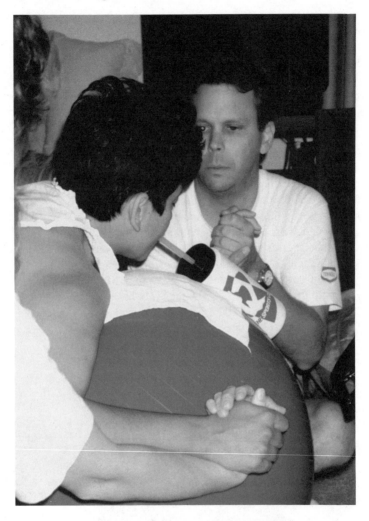

Drinking juice, water, and electrolyte balanced drinks
gives the mother energy and keeps her hydrated.

Chapter 11
Nourish the Body and Keep Moving

*The great thing in this world is not so much where we are
but in what direction we are moving.*
Oliver Wendell Holmes

By your endurance you will gain your lives.
Luke 21:19

In order for the mother's body to function effectively and for
her to deal with the pain of labor, she must be well hydrated and
have energy. Her nutrition or lack of it directly relates to pain
management. For that reason, many hospitals are now keeping
supplies of fruit juices, gelatin, popsicles, and electrolyte
balanced drinks for the mother's use during labor. Their aim is
for the mother to consume approximately 8 ounces and 120
calories an hour. It is not uncommon now to have the first
question asked of the labor mother upon entering the maternity
ward be "What type of juice would you prefer?." In birth centers
and home births, mothers are allowed to both drink and eat as
they desire, thus increasing their ability to cope with pain
through optimum nutrition.

Changing positions frequently is a very important labor
support technique. Changing positions frequently and utilizing
positions such as standing, walking, and hands-and-knees
stimulates the joint receptors which are large receptors that adapt
slowly but are also slow to habituate. Usually the mother does
this spontaneously. It is important to assess what is happening in
the labor when recommending position changes. Listed below are
some of the advantages and disadvantages of various labor
positions.

Standing

Advantages	Disadvantages
Excellent for oxygenation of the fetus	Unable to use with hypertension
Uses gravity	Unable to use with epidural anesthesia
Contractions are more effective	
Helps create a good pushing urge	
Can be used with hip squeeze	
Can be used with ice wrap	
Contractions are usually less painful	
Helps speed up a "poky" labor	

Walking

Advantages	Disadvantages
Less painful contractions	Unable to use with hypertension
Encourages uterine contractility	Telemetry needed if continuous electronic fetal monitoring is used
Baby well aligned in pelvis	Unable to use with epidural anesthesia
Excellent for promoting labor progress	
Good for back labor	
Encourages descent of fetus	
Can be used with ice wrap	

Stair Climbing

Advantages	Disadvantages
Combines gravity with slight changes in pelvic shape to encourage rotation of fetus	Unable to use with epidural anesthesia
Can be used with telemetry EFM	Telemetry needed if continuous EFM used

Sitting

Advantages	Disadvantages
Uses gravity	Unable to use with hypertension
Can be used with continuous EFM	Unable use with epidural anesthesia
Can be used with birth ball	
Works well in hospital beds	
Access to FHT's good	
May promote progress of labor	
Can be used with knee press	

Leaning

Advantages	Disadvantages
Helps rotate fetus	Unable to use with hypertension
Contractions often less painful	Unable to use with epidural anesthesia
Close contact with partner helpful	
Contractions often more productive	
Relieves back ache	
Facilitates use of counterpressure	
Can be used with continuous EFM	
Baby is well aligned in pelvis	
Can be used with hip squeeze	
Can be used with ice wrap	
May promote progress of labor	

Side Lying

Advantages	Disadvantages
Good fetal oxygenation	Access to FHT's difficult if mother is lying on same side as baby's back
Restful for mother	
Best position for hypertension	
Can be used with epidural anesthesia	
May make contractions more effective	
May promote progress of labor	
Can be used with knee press	
Can be used with heat or cold	

Squatting

Advantages	Disadvantages
Encourages descent of fetus	Tiring to the mother
May increase diameter of pelvis 2 cm	Difficult to hear FHT's
Assists in rotation of fetus	Unable to use with epidural anesthesia
Thighs keep baby well aligned	Unable to use with hypertension
Can be used with birth ball as support	

Hands and Knees

Advantages	Disadvantages
Helpful with bradycardia	Tiring to mother
Excellent for back labor	Unable to use with epidural anesthesia
Best position to rotate baby in persistent posterior presentation	
Takes pressure off hemorrhoids	
Excellent for back labor	
Counterpressure easy to use	
Most helpful when used with birth ball	
Pelvic rocking easy to do	

Stomp-Squat

For babies who are asynclitic (slightly crooked) in the mother's pelvis or for those mothers whose babies need to descend into the pelvis, try the stomp-squat. As the contraction starts, the mother stomps around the room similar to the way the elephant walks in the children's video *Jungle Book*. When the contraction reaches its peak, the mother squats for the remainder of the contraction. Via these stomping movements the baby is encouraged to change its position in the pelvis. The squatting increases the pelvic diameter and encourages the baby to descend. The stomp-squat-push, a variation of this technique, can be used in the second stage. The mother pushes at the peak of the contraction while in the squatting position.

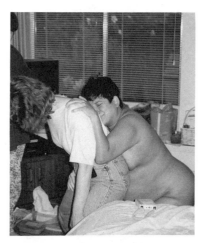 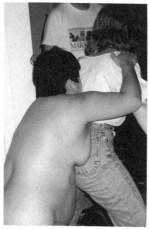

Stomp-squat and stomp-squat-push are techniques to help change the baby's position.

The squat bar on the birthing bed is another way of helping the mother squat if she must remain in the bed. If the squat bar is not available for the bed, the mother may still utilize this technique with the assistance of a person on either side of the bed for support. If the mother is not restricted in her labor positions, she might also squat on the floor beside the bed using the bed itself for support.

What About Back Labor?

Often the most difficult situation to deal with for both the mother and her labor support is the labor complicated by back labor or a persistent posterior position of the baby. This is where you will need to pull out everything you have in your "bag of tricks." At various points in the labor you will use the following labor support techniques: attention focusing, mental activity, counter pressure, the birth ball, the lunge, double hip squeeze, knee press, application of cold and heat, rolling pressure, tub or shower, slow dancing, dangle, walking, stair-climbing, hands and knees, pelvic rock, abdominal lift, and stomp-squat.

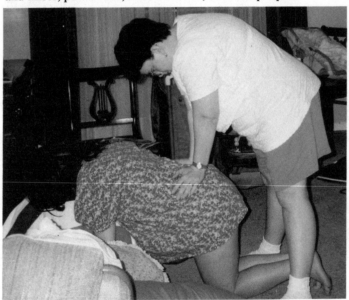

Constant pressure on the lower back called counterpressure
is a technique that benefits the mother who is experiencing back pain.

Counterpressure

Counterpressure is a technique that is applicable for those experiencing back pain. The mother's partner, nurse, midwife, or labor assistant applies constant pressure to the sacral area of the lower back. Simply ask the mother where she needs the pressure and how much pressure to apply. You may be surprised at the amount of pressure that the mother requests. When the mother asks for greater pressure, it is common to hear her be told "I'm pressing as hard as I can." Counterpressure can also be applied concurrently with the application of heat or cold.

At the End of the Rope

It is common for the mother to feel fragmented or panicky in transition or with a precipitous labor. When the mother hits a very low point, cries, is extremely tense, wants to give up, is in tremendous pain, or is temporarily unable to continue, use the panic routine, or as Penny Simkin calls it, the "take charge" routine.Touch the mother as it helps her feel grounded and less fragmented. At these times of panic you may notice that the mother has her eyes closed and is lost in the pain. Use a calm, yet "attention getting" tone of voice. The "take charge" or panic technique is as follows:

Remain calm.
Move in close to the mother so that you are face to face.
Anchor her by holding her tightly in your arms or
holding her face in your hands.
Tell her to open her eyes and look at you.
Remain calm and encouraging.
You may have to raise your voice to get her attention.
Your touch should be firm.
Tell her to follow you.
Breathe with her.
Pace her breathing with your hand.
Encourage her every breath.
Repeat phrases such as
You're OK
Breathe with me
That's the way

> *You've got it*
> *You're doing it*
> *Stay with me*
> *That's wonderful*
> *You're on top of it now*
> *Stay with it*
> *That contraction is going away*
>
> Change her rituals.
> Change her position.

Now that you have her attention and she is calmer, remind her that she is doing OK even if it doesn't feel OK. Talk to her between contractions. Ask her if what you are doing is helping. **Above all, remain calm; you are the foundation for her ability to get back in touch with her own strength and innate knowledge.** You will more than likely have to breathe with her and talk to her through each contraction for a while. Tell her that you'll stay with her and help her get through it. She will not remember what you say from one contraction to another so keep repeating what you say. When the contraction is over, tell her how well she did. Especially in the cases of precipitous labor, explain what is happening and its normalcy. Remind her of the marvelous job she is doing for her baby. The mother will require constant support and encouragement. Your constant support, encouragement and reassurance will help diminish her anxiety and fear of pain.

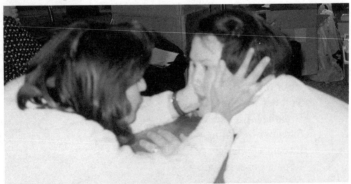

Along with the take charge routine, the mother will need constant
attention and support.

Do not give up on her. Remember that you are her anchor in a sea of pain and confusion. If you decide she can't do it, you are no longer able to help her. If you find you too have lost confidence, ask for help from another nurse, midwife, or labor assistant. Be sure someone reassures the father and family that the mother is fine and that this behavior is common.

Dealing with Failure to Progress

When dealing with "failure to progress," remember to use the following techniques: tincture of time, hands and knees over the birth ball, ambulation, undivided attention, massage, the dangle, the double hip squeeze, sitting on the birth ball, the "toilet trick," acupressure, reflexology, therapeutic touch, kneeling "frog style," slow dancing, , the lunge, hydrotherapy, music therapy, and the stomp-squat.

Pushing the Baby Into the World

During the second stage of labor, you may need to suggest position changes. Position change helps reduce the painful stimuli coming from pain receptors.

The following are the advantages and disadvantages of positions for the second stage.

Standing

Advantages	Disadvantages
Helps create a good pushing urge	Poor control at delivery
Use gravity for descent	Visualization very hard for birth attendant

Sitting

Advantages	Disadvantages
Uses gravity	May not be a good angle for those with a flat pubic arch

Sitting on toilet (the toilet trick)

Advantages	Disadvantages
Mother is used to open leg position & pelvic pressure in this environment	Edema from perineal pressure

Semi-sitting

Advantages	Disadvantages
Good visibility at delivery for mother	Access to perineum can be poor
Access to FHT's good Works well in hospital beds Can be good angle for those with flat pubic arch	Stress on perineum

Lithotomy

Advantages	Disadvantages
Stirrups support legs with heavy epidural block	Compression of all major vessels Laceration of perineum very likely No use of gravity

Avoid the lithotomy position unless no other position is effective.

Side-lying

Advantages	Disadvantages
Good fetal oxygenation	Need someone to help hold leg
Easier to relax between contractions	Mother may feel too passive
Lowers chance of perineal laceration Lowers need for episiotomy Access to perineum is excellent Partner can assist in delivery	

Squatting

Advantages	Disadvantages
Encourages rapid descent	Tiring to mother
Increases the diameter of pelvis	Sometimes difficult to hear FHT's
Requires less bearing down effort	Poor visibility of perineum
Thighs keep the baby well aligned	

Stomp-Squat-Push

Advantages	Disadvantages
Increases the diameter of the pelvis	Unable to use with epidural
Encourages rotation of asynclitic or posterior baby	Tiring to mother
Requires less bearing down effort	
Encourages descent	

Hands and Knees

Advantages	Disadvantages
Good for fetal bradycardia	Poor visibility for mother
Excellent visibility for birth attendant	Poor eye contact with mother
Useful with birth ball for support	Baby must be passed through mother's legs
Takes pressure off perineum	Can be disorienting to inexperienced birth attendant
Best position to avoid need for episiotomy	
Best position to avoid perineal laceration	
Excellent position for delivery of a large baby	
Best position to use for shoulder dystocia	

Encouragement during the second stage is a critically important labor support strategy. We should always pay attention to what we say and how we say it. As long as the mother is making progress and there is no fetal indication to accelerate the delivery process, continue to encourage the mother to listen to her own body and push as her body dictates. Praise her and encourage her efforts. For mothers with a flat pubic arch, you might suggest pushing on her back with her shoulders raised as it helps by utilizing the posterior part of the pelvis which is often roomier. This can also be accomplished with the mother side-lying and using her upper leg for leverage and support. When there is difficulty getting the baby under the pubic bone the following position is sometimes utilized as a last resort:

> Have the mother lie on her back with the head of the bed
> slightly elevated.
> Put her feet sole to sole and both feet with her hands
> As she pushes have her pull feet toward her.

Women with epidural anesthesia should not use this position.

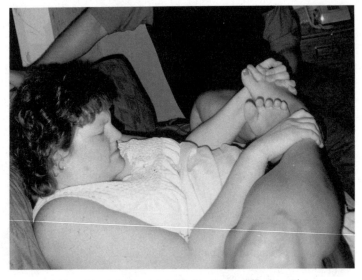

This pushing technique is helpful when there is difficulty getting
the baby under the pubic bone.

Pushing with an Epidural Anesthetic

Cheri Grant, a perinatal nurse and doula, has found the following technique helpful when the mother has an epidural anesthesia. When the mother is close to the second stage (dilatation of a rim or anterior lip) position the bed in a chair position and have the mother push three times lightly at the peak of a contraction only. With this technique, Cheri has found that by the time the mother reaches complete dilatation the baby is often at a +2 station.

Cheri has also developed a way for those women with a heavy epidural block to utilize gravity and an effective squatting position. She suggests the following:

> Put the bed in a chair position with the foot of the bed lowered and the stirrups (not foot pedals) attached to the bed.
>
> Put a bath blanket or pads inside the stirrups.
>
> Have the mother sit on the very edge of the top portion of the bed putting her arms in the stirrups.
>
> Position the mother's legs in a squat position.
>
> With a contraction, have the mother put her weight on her ams and hold herself up with the strength of her arms as she pulls her bottom slightly off the edge of the bed.
>
> Assist the mother in positioning herself back on the edge of the bed after each contraction.

Remind the mother to keep her perineum relaxed. The use of warm compresses is extremely helpful at this point as it increases the blood flow to the area, assists the perineal tissue in stretching, and feels good. You might prompt the mother to use the time in between contractions to get her energy back. The use of visualization is indicated in this situation. Suggest that the mother visualize her baby coming closer to her arms. A mirror, so the mother can see her progress, will help some mothers focus on pushing. Other mothers receive a tremendous boost of energy when they reach down and feel the baby's head as it is crowning. This can also help them push gently as the head delivers to avoid lacerations. At the delivery of the head it may be useful to have the mother push gradually, only in between contractions, and let the uterus do the pushing during a contraction. Remember that prolonged breath holding is not recommended unless rapid delivery is critical or the mother has no pushing urge due to a heavy epidural block.

Physical therapists warn that extreme caution should be used with pushing positions when the mother has epidural

anesthesia to avoid permanent damage due to the body being in anatomically stretched positions.

Talk to the Mother During Delivery

Pushing the baby into the world is hard work and it helps immensely if the mother is given constant encouragement. The following are tips for encouraging phrases to use during the delivery of the infant.

Drop your shoulder and your jaw.

With an open mouth, say ah-h-h-h (this prevents pushing too forcefully and helps avoid lacerations).

Reach down and feel your baby.

Let your baby out slowly.

The burning sensation is your body's way of saying, "Slow down, easy now."

Relax your bottom.

Reach down and bring your baby up to yourself.

Talk to your baby.

Dry your baby off.

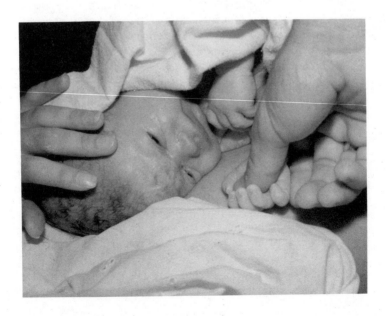

Chapter 12
Implementing Labor Support Strategies At All Birth Sites

Do not be afraid, but speak and do not be silent
Acts 18:9-10

Never doubt that a small group of concerned committed citizens
can't change the world....
Indeed it is the only thing that ever has.
Margaret Mead

Any technique can become a static one-size-fits-all prescription
that doesn't exactly fit anyone.
Aileen Crow

If you have faith as a mustard seed,
you will say to this mountain,
"Move from here to there: and it will move
and nothing will be impossible for you.
Matthew 17:20

The introduction of these labor support tools and techniques has already begun in maternity wards throughout North America. Without the knowledge of the techniques in this book, the only support tools caregivers have had to offer the laboring mother have been pharmacological ones such as IV narcotics and epidural anesthesia. With the use of labor support strategies such as the ones you have just read about, the mold of having the mother labor in bed, strapped to machines, tubes and wires, is being broken. Instead, nurses and professional labor assistants with the support of midwives and physicians are able to offer the laboring mother a myriad of options for coping with both labor and labor pain therefore decreasing her need to turn to pharmacology for pain relief.

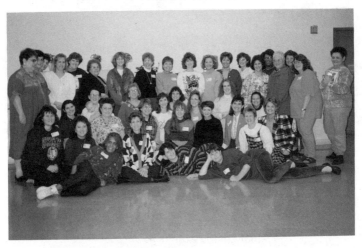

These hospital nurses and professional labor assistants are using
the support tools and comfort measures found in this book.

As with any change, implementing the strategies in this book
will require commitment and patience. Working together can
ease the burden on each of us individually. Expect resistance as
transformational change always meets with added resistance as it
involves a completely new way of looking at ourselves and our
world. Encourage critical thoughts and negative feedback. It will
show others that you too are willing to change.   Anticipate some
difficulties and learn to adapt what you have learned to your
specific environment. Be prepared to provide a context in which
others can understand the intent of the anticipated change.
Encourage communication both with other healthcare
professionals and the women you care for. Leave behind you a
birth environment that is nurturing to caregivers as well as
birthing women.   Believe in yourself and have the courage to use
this information to take new steps into uncharted territory.
Support other like-minded caregivers and stand together in the
task of providing a brighter future for childbearing women.

Instead of relying on narcotics and anesthesia as first line
coping tools, I urge you also to be innovative and begin using
these labor support tools and comfort measures as your first line
of defense against labor pain as have the nurses, midwives and

professional labor assistants at many birth sites throughout North America. Be a mentor for others by teaching them these new skills and strategies. As you work to help change the face of maternity care by using the techniques and strategies explained in this book, keep either the book or the convenient labor support reminder cards handy for reference. Adapt this material to the needs of each laboring woman.

Conscious, creative risk taking is the foundation for most personal as well as professional growth. Take the risk of empowering not only yourself but others as well. Empowering others is noble work as well as a different way of working together. Empowerment is not a "quick fix" but a way of helping women have the strength for the long haul, whether that be in birth or another journey in the road of life. We must be willing to take the risk of giving up power and control over others to gain higher motivation and loftier goals that afford us the opportunity for more fulfillment. Empowering others helps them to take responsibility for themselves as well as their actions and decisions. Empowerment enhances our work and liberates our creativity. It offers us the opportunity to look at the entire landscape rather than only a glimpse of the picture. Empowerment gives us the freedom to explore other avenues in our lives. It helps us each to use our talents to their fullest capacity. As you work toward implementing the labor support strategies, tools and techniques in this book, always remember that you are the backbone of our maternity care system and your wisdom and strong, yet gentle support will help change the portrait of birth that each mother paints for herself to include strokes of confidence, courage, power, strength and dignity.

Life is not a having and a getting.
But a being and a becoming.
Matthew Arnold

THE MENTOR'S SMILE

WE SHARE A MOMENT ALONG
LIFE'S WAY.
WE SHARE SO MANY
IT'S HARD TO SAY.

WHO WILL TOUCH OUR HEART
WITH A SMILE.
AND TOUCH OUR LIFE
FOR JUST A WHILE

INSPIRING US TO LIVE
OUR SPECIAL CALL.
TO REACH OUT TO OTHERS
AND GIVE OUR ALL.

HELPING THEM OBTAIN SOMETHING
OF UNMEASURABLE WORTH.
A MOST REWARDING AND
UNFORGETTABLE BIRTH.

ONE THAT WILL BRING DOWN
THROUGH THE YEARS.
NOTHING BUT MEMORIES OF
LOVE AND JOYOUS TEARS

AND THEY'LL NEVER KNOW
THE ONE WITH WHOM
THEY OWE MUCH OF THEIR
THANKS TO, IT'S YOU.

THE MENTOR WHO GAVE
ALL SHE COULD
TO HELP OTHERS THAT
EVENTUALLY WOULD...

TOUCH OTHER HEARTS
AND ALL THE WHILE,
THEY'RE SHARING WITH THEM
THEIR MENTOR'S SMILE.

BY LISA COX, WILLIAMSTON, SC

Resources

For more indepth information on many of the topics mentioned in this book, refer to the following material:

Acupressure's Potent Points by Michael Reed Gach
Accepting the Power to Heal by Dolores Krieger
Active Birth by Janet Balaskas
Acupressure for Common Ailments by Chris Janey and John Tindall
An Easier Childbirth by Gayle Peterson
Aromatherapy and Massage by Christine Wildwood
Aromatherapy for Common Ailments by Shirley Price
Aromatherapy for Pregnancy and Childbirth by Margaret Fawcett
Birth as an American Rite of Passage by Robbie Davis-Floyd
Birthing Normally by Gayle Peterson
Childbirth Education: Practice, Research and Theory, by Francine Nichols and Sharron Humenick
Creative Visualization by Shakti Gawain
Easing Labor Pain by Adrienne Lieberman
Gentle Birth Choices by Barbara Harper
Healing Yourself During Pregnancy by Joy Gardner
Heart and Hands by Elizabeth Davis
Labor Support Forms: A Guide to Doula Charting by Cheri Grant
Massage for Pain Relief by Peijian Shen
Mothering the Mother by Klaus, Klaus, & Kennell
Obstetric Myths vs. Research Realities by Henci Goer
Pregnant Woman's Comfort Book by Jennifer Louden
Special Delivery, The Complete Guide to Informed Birth By Rahima Baldwin
Special Women: The Role of the Professional Labor Assistant by Paulina Perez
The Birth Ball Book by Jan Prinzmetal & Brian Shiers
The Birth Partner by Penny Simkin
The Mother-Friendly Childbirth Initiative by The Coalition for Improving Maternity Services (CIMS)
Therapeutic Touch by Delores Krieger
Therapeutic Touch Inner Workbook by Delores Krieger
Timeless Healing by Herbert Benson

The Nurturing Touch at Birth

Water Magic by Mary Muryn
Wise Woman Herbal for the Childbearing Year by Susun Weed

The following videotapes and audiotapes are also helpful:

Cloud Dancer by Philip Elcano (a)
Comfort Measures for Childbirth featuring Penny Simkin (v)
Gentle Birth Choices by Barbara Harper (v)
Intracutaneous Injection by Reynolds (v)
Rain Dance by Philip Elcano (a)
Special Women: How a Labor Assistant Makes Birth Safer, More
Satisfying and Less Costly, featuring Paulina Perez (v)

The above books and videos as well as the following labor
support tools are available from Cutting Edge Press. Visit the
website at http://www.childbirth.org/CEP.html

Bellows Pump for Gymnastik Birth Ball
Birth Bags
     Starter Bag
     Advanced Bag
     Professional Bag
Doula Brochure
Doula Superbill Invoice
Doulas Have a Caring Heart Tote Bag
Doulas Have a Caring Heart Tee Shirt
Gymnastik Birth Ball
Gymnastik Birth Ball Carrying Strap
Happy Massager™
Labor Support Reminder Cards
Hot Sox
Mini Massager™
New Client Registration Cards
Tee Shirts with embroidered inscription
     Doulas Have a Caring Heart
Tee Shirts with printed inscription
     Special Birth Memories

Tote Bags with embroidered inscription
A Caring Heart
Nurses have a Caring Heart
Doulas Have a Caring Heart
Tote Bags with printed inscription
Special Birth Memories
Special Birth Memories Tote Bag
Special Birth Memories Tee Shirt
Universal Ice Wrap

Order Form

Postal Orders: Cutting Edge Press, 415 Bauxhall, Katy, Texas 77450-2203

Fax Orders: (281) 492-7223

For information call: (281) 497-8894

Please send me a free copy of the Cutting Edge Press Catalogue. We are now accepting credit card payments.

Name:_____

Address:_____

City:_____State_____Zip____

Visit our website at http://www.childbirth.org/CEP.html